Pieces of Me

Crushed by Grief. Held by Hope.

A Collection of Poetry

By Cherie Pinheiro

@Grief – The Write Way

E-book: 978-1-326-02492-5

Paperback: 978-1-291-99769-9

Hardcover: 978-1-291-99768-2

Dedication

I dedicate this book to two angel sisters.

One held in my arms.
The other in my womb.

Mallory Kate.
Bethany Grace.

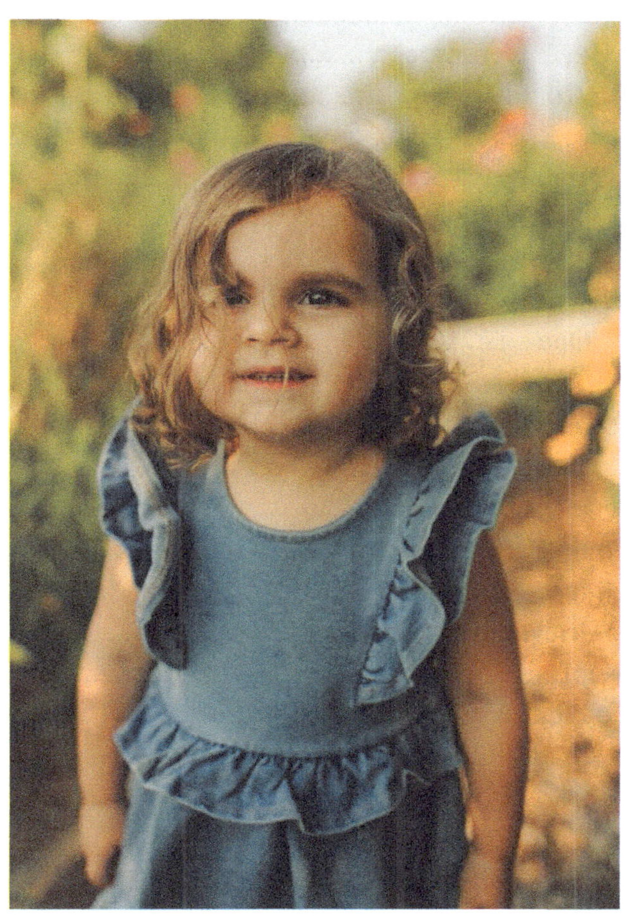

Table of Contents

Introduction

I don't think I've met one griever that wishes their loved one was never a part of their life. We all would choose the pain of losing our loved one over and over, again and again, over not having known them or loved them at all. No matter how short our time was together, no matter how long we now have to live without, we'd keep choosing the pain to have experienced the love.

The pain - there are days when the scream inside is so loud, that it feels not a damn thing can be done to silence it, or tone it down… even if just a notch. Days like these come more often than not in grief, and they are always the same. I do everything at first to resist or distract – everything I can possibly think of. I even resist talking to God.

But the big, bad grief is always stronger than I am. It huffs and it puffs and it blows my defenses straight down to the ground. While I resist, it persists. And its stamina can far outlast mine, eventually pinning my back up against the wall, leaving me no choice but to submit and surrender. Leaving me no choice but to look it in the eye and face it.

I don't like others around me when I feel like this. Not my husband. Not my kids. Especially not my kids. Not my trusted friends. Not my supportive family. No one! So I retreat and I isolate. I lie hidden in my own little bunker because conjuring the mask feels an impossibility. Faking the smile, too tall an order.

And I do the only thing that has been able to soothe the relentless ache of my soul since the start of this whole thing. I write. The hot, anguished tears roll off my cheeks while my belligerent words fill up countless blank pages once more. The pen to paper like water to a fire. As the words and the thoughts flow out, they extinguish the flames burning within me, and I get some sort of reprieve. At least for a little while.

This is the way it has been since I lost my youngest child in September of 2023 to a sudden and unexpected illness. It was 7 days total from the onset of her illness to her final breath, and I have been writing my way through this grief ever since. The Lord has gifted me with words, and I continue to pour my feelings out onto paper as a result.

I use writing as a way to make sense of this new world around me. I use writing to unscramble what's tangled up in my mind. I use writing as a way to conversate, draw close, and lament with God. I use writing as a means to remove the mask, to tell others what I need or don't need, and to somehow explain what's happening with me internally. I use writing for what I am unable to communicate verbally or show physically. I use writing to grieve.

Never in a million years did I think I'd publish a diary-like book of poetry confessing the intricate and intimate emotions of the most traumatizing experience of my life. Never in my life did I think I'd publish a second book, six short months later. But truly – that is grief in a nutshell. The unimaginable becomes real. My child, gone, is real. These books, born from the ashes, are real. The words keep coming because the grief does not stop. And I feel compelled to share them because I have a heart for other grievers. I want them to feel seen, heard, and understood through my words.

This book, *Pieces of Me*, is a sequel to and continuation of my first book, *I Will Speak of You*. It is a collection of poetry chronicling the depth and breadth of life after loss. Each poem is rooted in love and anchored in faith. Both these things, again, are not as simple as they seem. You will see love take on many different faces. You will see a faith that is both challenged and clung to. You will see grief pulled to the rawest corners of a shattered heart and hope held onto by the thinnest of threads. All of this is shared without filter to make grief, and all it comes with, visible and validated.

Before continuing on, it is important to know how this book has been structured. All the poems are placed in chronological order. Along the way of grieving and writing about one child, I dared to hope for another. And there was a moment in time where that very wish came to fruition. While I knew a new baby could never replace the child that I lost, I could not help but let some joy back in. I could not help but feel excitement for the future and a hope for tomorrow with this new chapter. To see with my own eyes this rainbow after the storm, to fill my home again with the noises of a baby, to get another chance… well, it felt like another dream taking shape.

But my other chance… my hope on the horizon… turned into heartbreak and hell. I lost that pregnancy, that rainbow baby. And that storm, combined with the storm I had already been in, sent me to a very dark and angry valley of grief. This was a pain I could not purpose. Choosing the pain over and again to experience the love just did not fit here.

I share all this so you understand the flow of the book. As you are reading the poetry, you will stumble upon *Section II - Pardon the Interruption.* This interruption is the writing that rose from the ashes of that pregnancy loss. The interruption ends with the start of *Section III.*

Thank you for taking this journey with me. It is true what they say about grief – it needs to be witnessed. And I have the utmost gratitude for anyone who stands in observance of mine through these pages.

Section I

Mallory Kate Pinheiro was born on April 2, 2021 at 5:20 p.m. She weighed 6 pounds 12 ounces and was 20 inches long. Every little feature was pure perfection, but there was one marking on her that caught my attention instantly. She came out with a good amount of very dark hair, but on her right side, and very visible, was a definitive streak of gray. I can remember asking the pediatrician about this streak, wondering if this patch of hair would darken to match the rest. He told me that it would not. He told me that it was kind of like a birthmark, and that as she grew older, this streak of hair would become even more pronounced.

Well, he was absolutely right. As she grew, this one of a kind physical characteristic was one of her defining features. It turned from gray to blonde as she got older, and it just made her as cute as can be, especially since it lay within a full head of gorgeous, bouncy, dark curls. Everyone she came across noticed it, commented on it, and just loved it.

I look back on that unique physical characteristic and see it as a sign that God had let me borrow one of His angels. Scripture even tells us in Proverbs 16:31. Gray is a crown of splendor; it is attained in the way of righteousness. I have no doubt that was God's marking on beautiful Mallory. His way of setting her apart from the rest. His way of intricately marking her righteousness at birth. She was sent with eternal intention. She brought our entire family to His light.

Mallory, I thank God every single day for choosing me to be at the center of your world from beginning to end. You are His gift that keeps on giving, and I cannot wait to see you again.

Dreamer

As a little girl,
I dreamed a big dream.
And it's not the kind
that one may glean.

I didn't dream of fortune,
or riches or fame.
I wasn't after notoriety,
or to make myself a name.

My dream was on that
of a grandeur scale.
I dreamed of "the happy"
of a fairy tale.

There was no future
brighter for me,
than the dream I dreamed
of a family.

Meeting true love
and saying "I do."
Growing our family
beyond just us two.

I had it all
in the palm of my hand.
I dreamed a big dream,
and it all went as planned.

You never would think
when your dreams come true,
that something will come along
and rip it away from you.

As I stared at the pieces
of my once upon a time,
I dreamed a new dream
for this family of mine.

I still don't desire riches
or fortune or fame.
I dream to make you
a household name.

So I create and I share
on a grandeur scale,
so all will know what happened
to my fairy tale.

I'll work this new dream,
I'll see it on through,
'til the whole wide world
learns about you.

Yes, I have this new dream.
and it's all about you.
This dream I dream,
it's built upon you.

Beautiful Classic

I rewatch your life like a movie.
I watch it again and again.
And every single time that I see it,
I beg for a different way to end.

The end doesn't fit with your storyline.
Where is your happy ever after?
If only I could rewrite the plotline,
and give you the ending sought after.

But even knowing the ending,
I still watch again and again.
Because even though I know where it's going,
it takes me back to where it began.

It's a heartbreaking but beautiful classic.
I watch and recite every line.
This tale of an angel on borrow,
who was mine once upon a short time.

My Garden of Grief

I have a beautiful garden,
and it's not the kind you think.
It's a different kind of garden.
It's a garden grown from grief.

The seeds were planted not long ago,
but the roots, they go down deep.
The roots are anchored in a love,
for a person I could not keep.

Others who pass my garden by,
don't get my garden's needs.
As from the outside looking in,
they see an unkempt mess of weeds.

"You see that part over there,"
they say…
"It's bushy and overgrown…"

I'll leave it as it is,
I thank.
It's meant to be as shown.

It's overgrown and it's bushy,
to make a kind of shade.
It gives me a place of solitude.
Aloneness is its' name.

"But how bout that flower over there.
This plant… it blocks the light.

It looks wilted and so droopy.
It looks a sad, sad sight."

Well that's because it is, I say.
You identified the name of that flower.
It's a beautiful bloom of sadness,
and it's meant to droop, NOT tower.

"And what about over there," they say,
"just stems, without any bloom.
Remove those dreary, bud-less flowers.
They look like doom and gloom."

Those ones I call hope.
And I know that they will grow.
They were germinated in a love.
When they're ready, buds will show.

Come on with me, I grumble.
I'll show you all the rest.
My grief cultivated this garden,
so I can explain it best.

These ones are perennials.
They'll come again each year.
These ones I call joy
because they remind me who was here.

And those annuals over there.
They sprout for damn good reason.
Named shock, guilt, fear, and anger.
Annuals stay for just a season.

And that beauty over there,
the red rose with the sharp thorn…
It pricks… when it's picked.
Pain… from a love born.

This is my garden –
my garden grown from grief.
It may look disorderly to you.
But to me, I know every leaf.

"This garden that you have,
it's like nothing that I've seen.
It's actually very beautiful
now that I know what it all means."

Well thank you, I reply.
But you never should have judged.
For every weed and every flower
are grief grown from love.

Thought you should know… This poem was a gift to another grieving mother. She, like me, shares the real and raw heartbreak of her loss in a public forum. The name of her page inspired the name of this poem. She has become a friend and a confidant, a sister in grief and a sister in Christ. Grief needs a village. Both of us have created one and have become a part of each others.

Different Narrative

I just want to wake up to a different narrative.

I want to wake up to a different story
but still remember every vivid detail of this one.

I want to remember the heartbreak,
the emptiness…
the never ending black hole.

I want to wake up thinking I'm still in the nightmare.

Then…
I want to be startled,
one by one,
by the old familiar things.

First startle –
your voice coming faintly from your room.

I'd ignore it at first,
thinking my mind is just playing tricks.

But then I'd hear it again -
a little bit louder,
a little bit more distinct.

I'd tip-toe to your room,
gently nudge the door a little bit open,
just enough to peek my head through.

Second startle –
the sight of you.

"You're here!" I'd exclaim.
You'd greet me with your beaming smile.
I'd frantically call to all the others,
who one by one
come into the room
to greet you.

Third startle –
no one is surprised.

And then it would hit me.
"It never happened," I'd whisper.
"It was all a bad dream," I'd rejoice.

But I'd always remember.

I'd save a space inside of me for all of that pain…
so I could never again,
take a single living moment,
with you,
with anyone,
for granted.

Failure

You don't easily forget the face of death.
Especially when,
you personally
watched it
unfold.

People don't forget that my child died.
But do they remember…
I watched her die.

I'm not talking about a final breath moment here.

I am talking about the life
that I saw
seep out of her
like air from a balloon,
over the course of a few days.

One by one,
I watched,
helplessly,
as organ after organ
shut down
and failed
on my child.

Minute by minute,
I watched,
as every measure possible
was taken
to sustain
her life.

Every measure possible –
without success.

Never before
had I understood
the true miracle of life –
the fragility of life.

How every little part of the whole matters.
How it all can change in an instant.

I will never unsee what I witnessed.
And I will never,
not ever,
be the same person again.

I don’t want to…

I don’t want to face another day without you.

Not one more day
bleeding into one more night,
bleeding into one more day,
without you.

I don’t want to find another purpose.

I don’t want to seek new meaning, or answers.

I don’t want to muster up anymore smiles,
fake any more pleasantries,
or show up to another damn thing –
without you.

I don’t want to.

Why can’t I have a say
on whether or not
I face another day.

Why can’t I be the one
to say,
“Lord, that’s enough…
I’m done.”

Betrayed

The ultimate betrayal –

When your heart stopped beating,
but mine ticked on.

When your lungs stopped breathing,
and mine breathed on.

The only way I make it through,
is to know my heart –
it beats for you.

The only right next thing to do,
Inhale. Exhale.
Breathe –
for you.

Best You Could

"You did the best you could
with the information you had at the time."

This is what they tell me.

But still…
I feel so damn guilty.

Plus how do they know?
They weren't there.

I could've done better.
I should've done more.

And the shame…
it has settled,
deep down in my core.

I carry this cross,
each and every day.

And to tell me I did my best,
well it just doesn't feel that way.

But I thank you,
for believing that so.

I pray your words take root,
and that one day, I'll be able to say,
"I know."

Tear ducts

The tears,
they fall like rain
for all the others.

Sobs,
they convulse out
like shockwaves
for all the others.

Person after person,
day after day
cannot look directly my way.

Not without wetness
puddling their eyes.
And little rivers
running down their sides.

But not me.
Not me.

It's like my ducts formed
their own little dam.
A barrier built –
where the tears could all cram.

And I return their gaze,
with a stone-like face,
accept their condolences
with an expressionless face.

.

But at day's end,
without a soul in sight,
the flood gates break open,
and I howl all the night.

“Things can always be worse…”

“Right?”

How many times have I heard that?
How many times have I said that?

To others.
To myself.

And the response –
always the same.

“Yep, it could always be worse.”

But not this time.
No, not this time.

This is as bad as it gets.

What is the reason?

What is the reason you were taken away?
Is it because I wasn't good enough?
Is God making me pay?

What is the reason you had to suffer so?
Was it to bring me to my knees?
So I'd beg you to go?

What is the reason to why you weren't healed?
Is there some lesson I should be learning?
Will it ever be revealed?

What is the reason for being dealt this brutal hand?
Was it to knock me off my feet
so I never again could stand?

What is the reason?
Will an answer ever suffice?
Oh what is the reason,
your love came at this price?

Dream Visit

Every night when I close my eyes,
I beg the Lord to hear my cries.

To help me through another day,
a dream visit is what I pray.

And not just any old kind of dream,
but one that feels as real as it seems.

You know the kind I'm talking about,
when you know they are with you
beyond a shadow of a doubt.

These vivid visits,
are not all the same.
But they keep us moving,
in grief's hard game.

Sometimes these dreams,
are just a voice.
Their unmistakable sound,
that makes your heart rejoice.

Other nights,
No peep. No sound.
But there they are…
just hanging round.

Exactly where they're supposed to be,
in the mix of it all… for all to see.

In these dreams,
we know it's a treat,
and hold onto the moment…
savor the sweet.

But after a while,
we're stirred awake,
and the pain sets in –
that familiar ache.

We close our eyes,
and will our mind,
to go back to that dream
for just a little more time.

But it never works,
the moment's passed.
So we jot it all down,
while the memory lasts.

"Thank you, Lord."
for the answered prayer.

Then a whisper to you…

"Again, tonight,
I'll meet you there."

"I'm sorry for your loss..."

Because what can I even say.
All the words,
they just fall short.
How can I possibly convey??

I can tell you
that when I heard the news,
my heart completely tore in two.

I can tell you
when your world stood still,
I felt it too,
my bones did chill.

I can tell you
that I feel the pain.
That it courses on through me,
that it seeps through my veins.

Yes, when I say I'm sorry,
it encompasses all of these things.
It means I hate your new world.
And I detest what grief brings.

But I know ALL of my words,
and ALL of my feelings
are NOTHING compared
to your daily dealings.

And there's no proper words
for me to convey,
that I am just so, so sorry,
your world is this way.

My Plus One

Thank you for inviting me,
even after all this time.
Thank you for inviting me,
though I consistently decline.

Thank you for inviting me.
Sometimes I think, "I'll go."
But as the hour draws nearer,
I know that I won't show.

Who would really want me there?
Have you really considered that?
I feel like the moment that I'd enter,
the lively party would turn flat.

Like I'd suction out the fun…
Be an eyesore to everyone.
Because right upon my arrival,
they'd see my grief plus one.

You see,
The Grief, it comes out with me.
It won't just stay behind.
And at the most inopportune moments,
it wreaks a havoc in my mind.

Then I'm stuck in the middle of this party,
begging my plus one,
to hold tight just a little longer,
so we don't ruin all the fun.

But The Grief keeps tugging at my side,
and there's no place in sight for me to hide.

I find that I can't breathe.
And I'm desperate, oh so desperate, to leave.

I try to go unnoticed.
Sneak away without a sound.
But it's hard to do when you're an eyesore,
and so many others are around.

And then the questions just start flowing.
And I can see the pity in their eyes.
And I'm flustered with myself,
that I'm the party's big demise.

You see, that's why I say no.
I've tried this all before.
But because of my plus one,
I don't trust myself no more.

But thank you for inviting me,
even after all this time.

But I promise,
I'm doing you a favor,
keeping me,
and my plus one…
behind.

Pieces of Me

Since losing you…
loss has become a trend.
You were just the beginning
of a "lost list" that has no end.

I lost my dear sweet child.
And you'd think that be enough.
But the losses just keep coming,
each bringing a brand new tough.

I lost my sense of certainty –
that things would always work out.
Replaced with a veil of uncertainty –
all confidence now clouded by doubt.

I lost my sense of purpose.
For what reason am I here?
I lost all sense of direction,
a future now unclear.

I've lost people in my corner,
my very ride or dies.
They no longer know what to do with me.
I'm a stranger in their eyes.

I've lost interests and all hobbies,
because the old things don't suffice.
I've lost my inner spark,
my flavor and my spice.

I've lost my reliability,
because my mind is not the same.
There's a constant mental fog,
and information I can't retain.

I've completely lost my balance,
from stable to unsteady.
I've lost my lust for life,
and I never feel able… or ready.

I have trouble making decisions,
and endless physical aches.
There's nothing I do well.
I'm a plethora of mistakes.

I've lost my ability to connect.
I'm uncomfortable with all others.
I just want to rush on through this life,
incognito and undercover.

I've lost my focus.
I've lost my peace.
I've lost my ways
to find release.

And it all started with the loss of you –
the loss that paved the way,
to this road where I just keep on losing,
pieces of me… along the way.

Do you have any idea?

Do you have any idea
what it feels like to breathe
with a cement block
pressing down on your chest?

Do you have any idea
what it feels like to quiet
a mind that no longer can rest?

Do you have any idea
what it feels like to carry
the weight of the world
on your back?

Do you have any idea
what it feels like to long for
a person you can never get back?

Do you have any idea
what it feels like to live with
a heart that's been broken to pieces?

Do you have any idea
what it feels like to know
you have to die
to know what real peace is?

Do you have any idea
what it feels like to hope
in something you just cannot see?

Do you have any idea
what it feels like to cope with
losing a life that was grown within thee?

Do you have any idea
what it feels like to hold
this unrelenting, unwavering grief?

Do you have any idea,
how it feels to grow old with,
new days that don't offer relief?

Many of you know…
I very well know that you do.

Oh how I wish that you didn't know.
I wish that. Truly, I do.

Since Losing You

Since losing you, I'm a soul without a home.
Since losing you, aimlessly I roam.

Since losing you, the sun has lost its shine.
Since losing you, I'm simply passing time.

Since losing you, I've lost my inner spark.
Since losing you, I stay hidden in my dark.

Since losing you, I'm a magnet attracting pain.
Since losing you, I can only see grief's stain.

Since losing you, the world's a vacant space.
Since losing you, I don't belong inside this place.

Since losing you, you are where I want to be.
Since losing you, I've slowly been losing me.

A Glimpse

Today I caught a glimpse
of who I used to be.
Her laughter filled the room.
She seemed younger.
Lighter.
Free.

I couldn't take my eyes off her,
so confident and sure.
All before her world was tainted,
she seemed happy,
relaxed,
secure.

And I couldn't help but wonder,
who this girl would be,
if darkness hadn't grabbed her,
and tied her up to he.

Yes I couldn't help but wonder,
who this girl could be,
if her eyes hadn't shifted –
because of the trauma
that lives in she.

This tiny little glimpse,
it made me miss her so.
But I realize, although that girl is gone,
she still radiates a glow.

She has lines across her face.
And dark circles beneath her eyes.
But every day she gives…
she loves…
despite how her insides cry.

Her laughter is not as loud,
and her movements don't exude
that same kind of proud,
there's something different that has brewed.

You can tell…
life has grown her older.
There's a heaviness –
a weight upon her shoulder.

But she still moves with a kind of grace.
She still has an inner beauty –
that no darkness could erase.

And I realize,
that although I miss
who she used to be,
that maybe now,
she's who she's meant to be.

Beautifully broken.
Weathered,
yet refined.
A symbol to others,
a light to her kind.

Life will knock you way the hell down.
But she has shown,
no matter how dark it gets,
your inner shine
can always
be found.

Thought you should know... This poem was inspired by a very real internal wrestle. Who would I be if this tragedy never happened, if I didn't have to look at the world with this new lens? At the same time, there is an internal recognition that there is this inner shine, a glow that still radiates despite the darkness. And how beautiful is that. To be weathered, yet refined. Broken, yet together.

You Should Be Here

You should be here,
HERE –
beside me.

I shouldn't have to wonder –
who you'd be.
You shouldn't only be –
a memory.

You should be here,
in tangible form –
where signs and wonders
you didn't have to perform.

You should be here,
with a life so long.
Your spirit, WITH flesh
in a body so strong.

You should be here,
with physical touch,
surrounded by those
who love you so much.

If love was a remedy,
you'd never have gone.
You should be here, sweet love.
It's where you belong.

Through it

The only way through it is through it.
And while I know this to be true,
it paints a false illusion too.

When you go through something,
you expect to come out the other side.
When you go through something,
you expect an end to the ride.

But grief has no other side.
There is no end to the tumultuous ride.

Grief just "IS"
each and every day.
And we need to feel it,
confront it,
as we pave our new way.

The only way through it is to face it.
To live it,
to breath it,
rather than
fight
or evade it.

The only way through it
is to take grief by the hand.
See it for the love that it is,
and form a togetherness band.

Because really,
you and grief,
you're on the same side.
Partners for life,
since the day that they died.

Yes, this grief,
it's on your same side,
a symbol of love,
so wear it with pride.

So when they say,
the only way through is through,
I think what they mean
is to accept this new you.

Yes, when they say
the only way through is through,
it means embrace this grief,
because this grief is now you.

For My Grieving Husband

You need to know that I see you.
Your tossing and turning at night.
Your heavy you try hard to make light.

I know where you go
when you're nowhere to be found,
behind those closed doors
with that whimpering sound.

So many times,
I ache to come to your side –
to kneel down beside you
with my arms open wide.

But I know that you know,
I'm there.

And you know, that I know
this pain, that we share.

And there's nothing
that each of us can do.
To alleviate the heartbreak
we're both living through.

And so I respect your time
to grieve on your own.
To cry out in the dark,
to "just be…"
alone.

And instead –
I press my hands
against that closed door.

And I whisper
"I love you's"
as my eyes start to pour.

And one day I'll tell you,
when I feel that I can,
that I sat on the other side of that door…
as your biggest fan.

The beauty in the brutal?
It's truly been you.
The way our good Lord
has worked through you.

Your time's so intentional.
Your walls broken down.
The way you take on more
when I feel I may drown.

I've never loved you more,
as I do right now.

I get on through this…

Well…
because of you,
that's how.

But your grief…
Your pain…

It matters too.

And I want you to know,
that I never not see you.

Thought you should know… It is clear that this poem was written for my husband. It is a "thought you should know" for him. All the while he has been seeing me, I thought he should know that I see him too, respectfully standing outside his grief, but always in it with him.

If Heaven Had a Window

Written from a child's perspective

Lord, I have a little favor,
I'd like to ask of You.
Can you build a Heaven window?
Can it go inside my room?

If Heaven had a window,
and I just could take a peek,
I'd promise not to speak of it,
its' secrets I would keep.

I just want a little glimpse.
Its' mysteries safe with me.
Please give me a little window,
into this place I long to see.

I hunger for its comfort,
and I crave to catch a sight,
of the loved ones gone before me,
into Your glorious light.

If Heaven had a window,
and I just could have a view,
no one would have to know it.
It could stay between me and You!

And maybe with this window,
if it's alright with You,
every once in a while,
You'd let me climb on through.

I won't be a bother.
No one will know I'm there.
I won't cause an inkling of disturbance,
during the moments that I'm there.

Oh can Heaven have a window?
And perhaps a two-way view?
So my person can come knockin'
and give me visits too?

I PROMISE to tell no one.
I pinky promise swear.
So can I have that Heaven window?
It's my one and only prayer.

Thought you should know… Every now and then I like to write a poem from a child's perspective. The inspiration always comes from my children. Their words, their prayers, woven up into my portrayal of it. It is my gift to them to bring voice to their grief and childlike perspective.

Take the Picture

Stop and take that picture.
Because one day it might be,
the only living proof,
of a life that used to be.

Stop and take that picture.
Because you just never know,
if capturing that moment,
is the last one you'll have to show.

Stop and take that picture.
It doesn't take much time.
It may one day spark a memory,
of a moment that slipped your mind.

Stop and take that picture.
It may one day be a treasure,
a slice of time with a certain someone,
whom you love beyond a measure.

Stop and take that picture.
Don't miss this chance you see,
as you truly just never know,
if there will be another opportunity.

Stop and take that picture!
It's something you won't regret.
Yes, stop and take that picture,
so this moment you won't forget.

What a Wonderful World

How wonderful the world could be
if pain could be no more,
if hateful things did not exist,
and we never kept a score.

How beautiful this life could be,
if evil was wiped out,
if we could put our trust in worldly things
without the slightest trace of doubt.

How magnificent this world could be
if we broke down all our walls,
if we welcomed in and stepped on up,
and caught each other's falls.

How wonderful this life could be
if we stopped the blame and shame,
if we pointed our fingers towards ourselves,
because we are guilty of just the same.

How beautiful this world could be
if we could see through another's eyes,
if we could place ourselves right in their shoes,
and truly empathize.

How magnificent this life could be
if we really could forgive and forget,
if we could offer people second chances
and give them a true reset.

How wonderful this world could be
if no one had to hide,
if challenges were met with grace
and there were no secrets to confide.

How beautiful this life could be
if success wasn't measured by things,
if we truly, deeply loved thy neighbor,
and found victory in the peace this brings.

How magical this world could be,
if tragedy was no more,
no more suffering of any kind,
and no temptations that could lure.

I believe a world like this could be,
where we all feel like we win,
and it truly is an attainable dream…
if we just keep our eyes on Him.

Empty Cup

My cup – it's empty,
impossible to fill.
I go now on fumes,
with no desire or will.

There's no take a break,
or ways to distract.
The burdens come with me –
a constant attack.

There's moments of joy –
little drips in my cup,
but the moment I get them,
they're instantly used up.

As a griever,
there's just more on your plate.
And while the world feels faster,
you can't move at that rate.

You sprint to keep up,
yet you still lag behind.
And much of the "to do" list
just escapes your grief mind!

Running on fumes –
all day and all night.
Constant exhaustion –
with no end in sight.

My cup – it's empty,
but the obligations still mount.

My cup – it's empty,
yet I must still pour out.

"I don't know how you do it…"

I often hear them say.
As if I've been gifted…
with some super human strength.

"I wouldn't be able to survive, if it were my child."
And I wonder how I should take this?
As if my response has been seen as mild.

Smile and nod.
Nod and smile.
That's often my go to.

Because I haven't found
the proper words
to explain this through and through.

You don't know how I do it?
How I keep getting
through each day.

Well I don't exactly
have a choice
as the time just ticks away.

You wouldn't be able to survive?

I assure you that you would.
Because your lungs would breathe
and your heart would beat
if you stood exactly where I stood.

Am I less of a griever?
Because I present to you as well?

Because I don't display the entire landscape
of this living,
breathing,
hell?

Maybe that's how I do it,
if you truly want to know.
I show you the surface of my grief
and not the layers buried below.

But please…

I am not some tall tale hero.
With this super human strength.
I'm simply just a griever,
trying to go the length.

“What doesn’t kill you makes you stronger…”

This is far from true.
Let me just share
a little something with you.

The after effects –
they hide.
You cannot see them
from the outside.

There are days when I worry
I will drown amongst tears.

There are days I’m submerged
in anxiety and fears.

On the outside –
all can appear as norm.

But on the inside –
a monstrous storm.

I have no choice,
but to go on.

And having no choice
does NOT make me strong.

The nights grow darker.
The days grow longer.

And as the time marches on,
I just do not feel stronger.

The downpours have weakened me.
They have almost completely depleted me.

What doesn't kill you makes you stronger?

How about this instead…

I'm just barely breathing.
I'm like the walking dead.

Good Samaritan

She sat in hysterics,
the tears flowing down,
on a quiet park bench
with no one around.

But little did she know,
with each anguished tear,
the sounds of her crying,
drew someone else near.

"Ma'am, are you hurt?
Is there something I can do?
I've been wanting to approach,
but not be frightening to you.

Is there someone I can call?
Is there room there for two?
I can't just go on my way.
May I sit there with you?"

With barely a glance,
she shook her head no.
But the dear, sweet man,
he just couldn't go.

"I'll stay at this distance,
I won't come too near.
But I just can't go leaving,
you like this here."

For a long while,
she sobbed and she sobbed.
And then finally she screamed,
"I've been robbed. I've been robbed."

The man jumped to attention,
"Which way did he go?
Did you see what he looked like?
Tell me all that you know."

"No, no.
You don't understand.
I've been robbed of a life!
A future… my plan."

"I'm sorry, ma'am,
I don't know what you mean."
She threw her head in her hands
with an agonizing scream.

"I've been robbed,
I've been robbed,"
she continued to sob.

"And there's nothing you can do!
No mystery to solve.

I've been robbed of my child,
watching her grow.
I've been robbed of nurturing,
and loving her so.

I've been robbed of my purpose,
my direction, my place.
My identity stolen,
and it can't be replaced.

So much was taken.
And it can't be returned.
Her life. My life.
Set fire… and burned.

What's been stolen –
it has bled me bone dry.
Why was I left here?
Why?
WHY?"

And at that moment,
she looked at the man,
who was now sitting beside her
wiping his tears with his hand.

"So, no sir…
there's no one to call.
There's nothing that you can do,
to lift me up from this fall."

With that, she got up to go…

"Wait, young lady.
Not yet…
don't go!

I know there is nothing
that I can do,
but I'd like to meet your sweet child.
Get to know her… through you."

Fresh tears blinked out
her red-rimmed eyes.
She slowly sat down again,
with this man at her side.

She gently began
tale after tale –
from the end to the beginning,
her angel unveiled.

"I guess I was wrong,
thinking there was nothing you could do.

This is the best thing to offer,
allowing me to share her… with you.

Thank you sir,
for this gift of your time…"

"No no, dear lady…
The gratitude's all mine."

Thought you should know… This poem was inspired by a beautiful encounter with a man at the cemetery. He had shared that he had seen me at my child's tombstone and that he couldn't get me out of his mind thereafter. He came back looking for me every day, until our timing aligned once more. The two of us sat together, swapping stories and sharing tears for hours. I learned all of his wife, and he learned all of my Mallory. I was very moved by the good samaritan.

That is Grief…

I am grieving.

But what that looks like –
is constantly changing.

What it looks like in the morning –
shifts by the afternoon.

What it resembled yesterday –
is a stark contrast to today.
And God knows what it will look like tomorrow.

Last year looked nothing like this year.
And what felt right a minute ago,
doesn't feel so good right now.

But that is grief.

Constant fluctuations and mutations.
Constant instability and variability.

Every single feeling –
with its own little spark plug.

Each –
with the power to completely ignite.

And they feed off each other.
One catching fire from the other,
until all emotions are combusting at once.

Yes, that is grief.

Living with all these wildfires.
Breathing amidst all these flames.
Surviving this raging inferno,
one blaze at a time.

Death, Where is Your Sting?

The Christian way
is to sing and say,
"Oh death where is your sting?"

But I've met death.
Seen final breath.
And I'm left here struggling?

The truth is,
death has a sting.
And it hurts like hell
if you're wondering.

I know it's not
the final hold.
And that the sting of death,
will one day fold.

But while I'm stuck in this purgatory,
please don't expect I be celebratory.

Because the sting of death
burns through my flesh.
And it will singe and scorch,
'til my final breath.

Why you?

How come death
barged down your door?

Why attack innocence,
something so pure?

Why make a light burn out…
when so much evil lurks about?

Why take the good ones,
with no second chance?

Why allow the wicked ones
to repeat their same dance.

It doesn't feel fair.
It doesn't seem right.

Why extinguish the light
but keep the dark in sight?

This is the backwards kingdom.

But why is that so?

It should be right side up.
Just like the place we will go.

What's even the point,
of living in this space,
if for the duration of our lives
it's heaven we chase.

Why be in a world
we're not supposed to love?

Why give us these views
if we should set sights above?

Sometimes it all feels
like some cruel game.

Like we've been thrown to the wolves
and only the vile remain.

Our Lord, our God,
turn this kingdom around!

You have the power to do this.
We walk on Your ground.

I pray this to You, God.
Turn this kingdom around.

Cast light in the darkness…
Let Your goodness abound.

Thought you should know… This poem was inspired by the question every griever asks at some point. Why our person? Why God? There is so much evil in this world and it often feels like it's the "good ones" that don't get second chances. This poem exemplifies trying to make sense of that.

Take Me Back

Take me back
to those early days of grief.

When it was okay
to not be okay.

When it was okay
to not turn a new leaf.

Take me back
to the beginning of the after –

when tears were not hidden
or masked behind laughter.

Take me back
to when the world stopped turning –

to when the fog couldn't be lifted
and the fire kept burning.

Yes, take me back
to these earliest days –

where I could get lost in my thoughts
and stare at the blaze.

When did it shift –
what was accepted?

When did it lift –
the smog that protected?

When did obligations –
start to mount?

Who placed expectations –
that now do count?

Take me back
to those earliest days.

I need more time
to live in that haze.

Just take me back!
Stop this world turning.

I just can't go forward,
with my stomach still churning.

Yes take me back
to when the world stopped turning,

to when it still was okay
to dwell deep… in yearning.

Stepping Out or Staying In

Stepping out?
Or Staying in?
That seems to be
the big question.

Every time
I step out the door,
I come face to face
with what is no more.

Around every bend,
and every turn,
I see my heart's desire
and I suffer the burn.

It's so hard to go about,
avoiding these flames.
Envying the world.
and hiding my strain.

Sometimes it's easier
to hideaway,
to not step out
into the day.

No more small talk.
No acting okay.
No more reminders
of all you lost on that day.

It's probably easier,
on the world too,
to not have to constantly,
slam in to you.

You're a reminder to them
of what life can throw.
You're a walking example
of how the story can go.

And as time marches on,
and you still stay lost.
You become that bump in the road
to avoid at all costs.

Because the world doesn't want
heartache and strife.
They will stop for a moment.
But then go on with their life.

The world doesn't want
backwards moving.
They want forward progress,
making headway… improving.

So it's easier really,
to just stay in.
It's easier on you
and it's easier on them.

Malfunctions

Death has snipped away
the strings of my heart.

Leaving no possibility
to tug,
to pull,
to yank on its' chains.

Leaving no chance
to strike
a chord
of emotion.

So has it
blockaded
the ducts
of my eyes.

Tears –
shut in, and crowded.
Little rivers,
denied access,
to roll off the cheek.

Death has impeded
normal brain power.

Thoughts race.
Words don't retrieve.
Information does not file.

There's a constant fog
over the control center.
A literal wrench,
in homeostasis.

Death leaves a person faulty.
I… am faulty.

I have a detached heart –
that burns instead of beats.

I have eyes –
that sting instead of water.

And a mind –
that clouds instead of clears,
that drifts instead of drives,
that's failing instead of functioning.

I am broken.
I am broken.

Not Her

Who was I
before grief broke down my door?
I don't even recognize me
anymore.

If she passed me,
on the street,
would I know her?
And her know me?

Or would she not
even glance my way,
with nothing nudging her
to stop and say, "Hey..."

Not a thing that's familiar
to heighten her sense.
She never would think
"I'm her" in past tense.

And perhaps that's why
we don't know,
all that lies
in our tomorrow.

Because if we did,
who'd want to go!
Not her, I mean me.
Not willingly. No.

Worthy

I feel so unworthy –
of this beat in my heart,
this air in my lungs,
waking to a new start.

I feel so undeserving –
of my feet on these grounds,
my hands in this air,
all these sights and these sounds.

I feel so undeserving –
of the wind at my back,
my face in the breeze,
these years to keep track.

Why do I get –
days of blue skies,
sunrises,
sunsets,
mountain views, ocean tides.

Why am I worthy –
of all the moon's phases,
the changing of seasons,
and the nighttime stargazing.

Why do I deserve –
to follow a dream,
to set lofty goals,
to release and redeem.

The truth is…
I'm unworthy of worth,
completely underserving
to walk on this Earth.

But you know who is deserving
of sunshine so bright?
Of entering new days?
And shutting down a new night?

You know who is deserving
of a steady, drumming heart?
To breathe in and breathe out,
and wake up to new starts?

You know who is deserving
of moon phases and seasons,
sunrises, sunsets,
early mornings, late evenings?

You know who does deserve
ocean tides, mountain views,
new dreams, new goals,
and skies oh so blue?

It's you who is worthy.
It's you.
YOU.

Entangled Webs

Entangled webs –
define,
and redefine,
who I am.

And I can't help but wonder,
who I might be,
if these knots were untangled,
unwoven, set free.

Would I stay caught and entrapped?
Because they're rooted in me?
Or would I finally be liberated…
unshackled, cut free.

Would I stay who I am?
Or would I finally see,
the person I envisioned,
who I always dreamed,
I could be.

Pencil to Paper

I've got all these thoughts,
swirling in my brain,
thrusting this way and that way,
driving me insane!

And the only way,
I can steer them out,
is to bring pencil to paper,
while they frenzy about.

The words gush out,
unleashed from their cage!
And they scrawl something furiously,
across that blank page.

CAPITALS for emphasis.
Punctuation to breathe,
an aching hand,
giving the heart a reprieve.

The brain stops swirling.
The mind stops to race,
as my thoughts take stride
with my pencil's pace.

With steadied breaths,
the pencil drops down.
It's mission accomplished!
A storm now sound.

And it's not 'til after,
when I read it all back,
that I make some sort of sense
of my grief brain attack.

I take in the words,
wondering how it could be –
that the thoughts on this page,
were written by me.

Thought you should know… This poem was inspired by what it feels like every time I write a new piece. Most of the time I don't even know what I'm writing about or dealing with until I've finished and have read it on over. I often find myself taken aback by my words, not sure how I produced what I did. Writing truly is how I make sense of grief and how I'm feeling. I am very grateful to the Lord for giving me this mechanism to cope, both for myself and for others.

I will keep on sharing…

More often than not I question why I am sharing.

Why does the world need to know this –
my inner most thoughts,
my deepest, darkest, pain.

And the simple answer is they don't.
They don't need to know any of it.

They don't need to know
the anguished cries of my soul.

They don't need to know
the unrelenting and repeated what ifs,
or the way my worries paralyze me with fear.

They don't need to know
the sleepless nights,
or being jolted awake
by nightmarish images.

They don't need to know how friendships
and family ties have changed,
how I feel like an outsider
wherever I go.

No, no one needs to know about any of that.

And I get real close to throwing in the towel,
to muting the sound of my voice to the outside world.
Forcing myself to be quiet.

But every single time…
Every… single… time…
This eensy-weensy little voice whispers in my ear.

"What if there is one person who does need to hear it?
What if there is one person who does look for it every day,
who needs it –
counts on it –
to know that what they are feeling is okay…
normal even.

What if you don't even know who this person is,
like they are just this little fly on the wall,
listening… always just listening… and resonating.

They don't have the words that you do.
And they can't find their voice to respond.

But they are there.

Feeling seen.
Feeling heard.
Feeling validated."

And these what ifs marinate in my mind.
They sing a sweet melody to my soul.

"Well then I will keep on sharing…" I answer.
"I will keep on sharing."

Another Year Gone

Sometimes I just look at your picture,
and whisper…

How the hell are you not here?

How have the days
turned to weeks
and then months.

How have the months
turned into a year.

And now
another year has gone.

How could this possibly be?

Gone the same time as I had you,
Heaven –
holding you longer than me.

It all feels so wrong.
That in equivalent time,
one can feel short,
and the other so long.

I miss you my angel.
You're where I should be.
I need you sweet angel.
Heaven – come get me.

"She is always with you"

Let me ask you this…

Would you want your loved one
to be "with you"
in the same way
mine is "with me…"

I didn't think so.

Thought you should know… This is something that so many tell me. And I know it comes from the most loving place. But it is a hard one. I want my child here with me physically, where I can see her, and feel her, and hear her, and love on her. I want her here in the flesh. When people tell me she is always with me, it does not provide the comfort that they think it does. I am missing my daughter. And she is not with me. She's in heaven. Sometimes, it is easiest for me to explain how these platitudes come off by turning them back on the person. It is not to be mean or rude, but it is to make them think. An attempt to help them understand.

New believer

I have this insatiable appetite.
Hungry –
for no one but You.
Please feed me more of Your word, God.
It's like I'd been starved
before I'd met You.

Your words satisfy my cravings.
They nourish my soul that needs saving.

Their richness is making me alive.
I am no longer failure to thrive.

Your word,
like the milk of a mother.
It's fullness –
growing me,
like no other.

Available right on demand.
A force in the palm of my hand.

It knows exactly what I need.
Power in each and every feed.

And as the fruitfulness courses on through,
I am a new creation.
The old me passes away,
and I'm born again…
made new.

It’s You

People don’t know how I do it.
But it’s not me.
It’s You.

As from the moment
my world darkened,
Your light came shining through.

You whispered me
Your promises.
And in my soul
they’re now ingrained.

They filled me with a calm,
the kind that cannot
be explained.

Your words –
they planted seeds.
And new roots began to sow.

Your words –
removed my weeds.
And a new me began to grow.

I’m no longer scared of rain.
The sun will sure break through.
I trust this… well because…
my eyes are fixed on You.

Whatever comes my way,
I know I'm not alone.
Because Your walking right beside me
'til the day You bring me home.

Thought you should know… This poem was written on June 22nd 2025, two days before my second trimester miscarriage. I wrote this poem, lying in bed, before I closed my eyes for the night. It was a love letter to the Lord. It was a praise report, acknowledging that I am where I am because of Him and that I could get through anything as long as I had Him with me.

Section II – Pardon the Interruption

On June 24th 2025, I went to the doctor for a regularly scheduled prenatal visit. I did my usual weigh-in and urine sample before following the nurse into the examination room. She squirted the iced cold jelly onto my belly, and I had my usual sarcastic response.

"What do you guys do, store this stuff in the freezer or something?" We both laughed as she began to move the Doppler around my lower abdomen. The seconds of scanning turned into several minutes. Suddenly, I had a sinking feeling.

"Uh oh…" I said.

"No, no," she reassured. "The baby is still really small, and it can be hard to detect sometimes. I'll send the doctor in to try." And she left the room.

I sent a message to my husband and said a quick prayer. Then I waited. And I waited. And I waited.

After about 25 minutes, the doctor came in with apologies for the delay. Round 2 of the cold jelly squirt was underway, and again the seconds turned into long silencing minutes as the doctor and I both listened for the sound we longed to hear, but with no avail.

On my walk to the room for the ultrasound, I sent another message to Brian, who quickly responded, "I'm on my way." I lay on the ultrasound table and braced myself for the third squirt of the iced cold jelly, but this time, I couldn't seem to feel the frigid temperature against the nerves crawling all over my skin. The technician turned the screen so it only faced her, and she scanned away while I tried to read her expression.

Without a word, she got up and left the room, returning seconds later with the doctor at her side. Again, she picked up the wand to scan across my belly, and the two had their eyes glued to the screen. I couldn't take the silence any longer.

"Please just tell me." I pleaded.

And they did tell me what my heart already knew. That at just 14 weeks gestation, my growing baby girl had died.

So much was wrapped up in this rainbow baby of mine. First and foremost, she was a symbol of trust and surrender to the Lord. I was beyond terrified to try again for another child after the sudden and tragic death of my daughter. I was terrified to have a child who was unhealthy. I was terrified to have another healthy child that at any second could turn ill. I was terrified to disrupt the "new normal" we had found in our home. I was terrified of every single unknown that my mind could muster up. But mostly, I was scared the Lord would say no, that He wouldn't trust me with new life when I had failed to protect a life He had already given me. I was terrified for confirmation that He had closed my womb, and quite frankly I was more comfortable with not trying and not knowing His answer, than trying and hearing a hard no.

I refused to let go of this little piece of control for a very long time. The thoughts of growing our family would swirl in my mind on the regular, and I would do all I could to push those thoughts out of my mind because the fear of the unknowns, and the fear of the "no" were just too much to wrestle with. I flat out ignored any of these spirit let stirrings. "You can have all of me Lord, but You cannot have the key to this one compartment."

Time in God's word, time spent in prayer, and messages heard at church kept bringing me back to this one very area that I just could not surrender. I felt so convicted that the Lord was telling me to trust Him with this. So I did. I let go and let God. And it worked. Not right away, but it worked.

This rainbow baby felt like a symbol of God's forgiveness to me, a symbol of my surrender to Him, a symbol of my love for Him, and His love for me, the cherry on top of a blooming and intimate relationship. This rainbow baby felt like another chance for our whole family – an addition to, and not a replacement of, the child we lost. I felt repurposed, like God really does have a plan for me, like He really is just and sovereign and all-knowing. For the first time since the loss of Mallory, I looked forward to tomorrow. I felt some excitement to look ahead.

This pregnancy loss was and is a very different loss from the loss of Mallory. But let me confirm that it does not feel inferior. There were so many hopes and dreams wrapped up in this new life. Another future blown up in my face. This loss left me feeling absolutely and completely crushed. Crushed physically. Crushed emotionally, and worst of all, crushed spiritually.

The writings that follow illustrate a very dark season of grief. My faith had been shaken. After Mallory died, God was the only person I wanted to talk to. I felt His presence and His love so strongly. I felt Him guiding my steps, directing my thoughts, giving me words. I knew He was the one who set limits to her time. It brought me to my knees, but not in anger. He saved her. He released her from the hell on earth that would have been her life had she survived. I looked past that He allowed sickness to enter her life and latched onto that He rescued her from a life of living with it. I became desperate to know Him. Desperate to know that I, too, could get to where she was.

And I made that the cornerstone of my new existence. Believing wholeheartedly that when He saved her, He also saved me. I continually showed my gratitude by growing in my faith. Deepening in my understanding. Surrendering. Trusting. Obeying. Transforming.

And then this…

I just felt so misguided. So let down. Like I was lovingly rebuilt just to be re-broken. The safe place that I went to after the loss of Mallory no longer felt safe. I couldn't look to the Lord in the same way that I had been. And all the writings that follow depict this. Unfiltered anger at God. Questioning His ways. Wrestling with His truths. Clinging to His hope while also wanting to turn my back on it.

I share it all because this, too, deserves a seat at the grief table. Am I trying to pull people away from their faith? Absolutely not. I AM a believer. And I would want nothing more than to lead people to rest in God's word, not stray from it. Yet these are real feelings, and I want to normalize them like all the others. They deserve to be validated and witnessed like all the rest. And if we are ever to fully rest in God's faithfulness and love, then we need to voice and confront these feelings so that we can work to release them.

Thank you for entering this dark season with me. Before you get started, let me introduce you to my rainbow baby. Bethany Grace is her name. Brian and I picked it out very shortly after we found out we were having a girl. Bethany is the village where Jesus raised Lazarus from the dead. It is also where He ascended into Heaven after his resurrection. And Grace… well, that is pretty self-explanatory.

It means kindness. It means mercy. It means blessing and beauty. And this rainbow baby was a much-wanted, answered prayer. We wanted her name to reflect our love and thanksgiving to the Lord. So, we chose the village where one of his most breathtaking miracles occurred. We chose the village where he ascended to the home we long for, the home that holds one of our children. And we chose Grace, as this new growing life signified His favor upon us.

Answered Prayer

I didn't think this was possible for me.
That the door was firmly shut tight.
That the Lord did not want this for me.
That I was unworthy of this in His sight.

I took the stance
that if it was meant to be,
the Lord would make it happen,
with no trying from me.

For if it's His will,
it's His will,
regardless of what I do.

So I just tried to "know"
and "be still,"
and His plan would surely shine through.

But in my wanting and waiting,
I came to a new revelation.

I heard the Lord say,
"I know what you need,
but in order to get it,
surrender to me.

You say that you have.
But we both know that's not true.
You've been holding back
the biggest piece of you."

I knew it was true.
But I still couldn't let go.
The "what ifs" and the worries,
I couldn't relinquish control.

But then came a day
after some time in His word,
where I read a message
of a prayer that was heard.

A woman who
was along in her years,
conceived a child,
with grateful tears.

I, too,
am along in years.
My age, a factor,
in controlling my fears.

But this message planted
a tiny seed
that all is possible
when you let the Lord lead.

And at that moment,
I looked out the window.
The rain met the sun
and formed a glorious rainbow.

I felt so strongly
the Lord speaking to me.
He said, "Let go, and Let God."
And I submitted to He.

And just like Elizabeth
favored in Luke 1,
I stand here in awe
of what the Lord has done.

He's gifted me life.
He has a plan for me,
a beautiful new addition
for my family.

Thank you Jesus.
There's life in your word.
I give You all the praise
for this prayer that was heard.

Thought you should know... I wrote this poem after I found out that I was pregnant with what would have been my rainbow baby. I wanted to capture this moment, not just the growing new life, but all the events that led to it. The wrestling. The fear. The prayers. The submission. The full surrender. I was in complete awe of the Lord when I saw those two pink lines. I felt so lovingly led to this exact place – like it was the culmination of the work He was doing within me since the loss of Mallory. To me this pregnancy was proof that God could work in any situation, that He only requires surrender.

Two Pink Lines

Everything changes
with those two pink lines.
An instant shift,
to the thoughts of your mind.

Excitement, angst.
Disbelief, joy.
The instant wonder,
if it's a girl or a boy.

Knowing it's early,
but a desire to share.
A hand on your belly,
in awe of what's there.

Time ticks slowly,
week after week,
while you await that first visit,
for the reassurance you seek.

You lower your pants,
lift up your shirt.
Nervous anticipation,
with the cold jelly they squirt.

You turn your head.
Eyes on the screen.
Up pops the most beautiful image,
that you've ever seen.

Tears sting your eyes.
You breathe a sigh of relief.
There's a growing baby!
You now can believe!

You announce your news.
Baby things you peruse.
You make sure you're on point,
with all the don'ts and the do's.

You brainstorm names.
You prepare a space,
while counting down
when you'll meet face to face.

But upon your next visit,
you never expect,
the crushing news
that awaits you next.

Your head is spinning.
And your heart starts to race,
as the doctor searches
for a heartbeat it can't trace.

You're sent back to that room,
of that first ultrasound,
where just a few weeks before,
a heartbeat was found.

But this time,
they turn the screen away.

Yet you can read their expression,
and what they're about to say.

They force their eyes
to look into yours.
"We are so, so sorry,
but your baby's no more."

They go over your options.
But you just can't comprehend,
as your mind is just swirling,
with how… and when???

And once again,
the emotions pour out,
as this new dream for your future,
just fades and bleeds out.

Rainbow Baby

There's so much wrapped up
in that rainbow baby of mine.

A true gift made of love –
nothing short of divine.

The sound of a heartbeat –
after another's has stopped.
A new chance at a life –
that so quickly was dropped.

The prayers with the tears –
in wishing this so.
The worry and fear –
that you had to let go.

Month after month –
of getting let down,
when two pink lines
were nowhere to be found.

But on that final month,
you were willing to try –
that rainbow…
that miracle…
that dream came alive.

There's so much wrapped up
in those two pink lines.

New hope.
New chapter.
New light to bring shine.

Oh rainbow baby,
how wanted you are!
The very wish
wished upon that star.

So what in the world
can one possibly do…
When that rainbow baby
goes to Heaven too?

Missed Miscarriage

A Missed Miscarriage –
That's what they call it.

A Silent Miscarriage –
That's what you were.

Silent because there were no symptoms.
Missed because nothing physically happened.

No spotting.
No bleeding.
No cramping.

No loss of pregnancy symptoms, at all.

Well that's not totally true I guess.
The nausea had lessened.
The energy had returned.

"Every pregnancy is different," they'd say.

But I know now that was a quiet whisper –
a warning missed.

Things were not going as they should.

The Note

If the Lord calls me home,
and it takes you by surprise…
I leave this here note,
as a way to say goodbye.

To my husband and best friend,
you are the love of my life.
The greatest gift you gave me
was the title of wife.

I never felt lost,
as long as I had you.
Every threshold we crossed,
we did it… me and you.

Thank you for loving me,
through good times and bad.
Thank you for giving me,
absolutely everything you had.

To my firstborn –
my son…
you gave me the best gift of anyone!
Thank you, sweet child,
for making me a mom.

Your sensitivity –
and loving heart,
captured mine,
from the very start.

Please remember,
when you think you can't,
you can!

And I'm always cheering you on,
as your biggest fan.

In fact,
you're exactly what I'd look for
in a fine young man.

To my first daughter, my girl,
my perfect little pearl,
so sassy, yet sweet,
who never skips a beat…

There's so much the same,
that we like to do.
Two peas in a pod!
Me…
and you.

You put yourself out there.
Never afraid of something new.
Two beautiful qualities,
I always admired in you.

I loved every minute,
of watching you both grow,
and you've made me the proudest mama,
I sure hope you do know.

My husband, my children –
my life's greatest prize,
please don't waste your time
trying to answer "the why's."

You already know –
no answer… will satisfy.

So I'll love you at this distance.
I will remain at your side.

Because truly you know,
my love –
it won't die.

Thought you should know… This poem was written from my hospital bed. I was in the hospital for two days as my body was ripened and prepped to evacuate a 14 week gestation baby. When the doctor spoke to me and my husband, he highlighted some risks that were possible, yet unlikely, with my procedure. The risk of my uterus being perforated. The risk of hemorrhaging and needing a transfusion. The risk of infection. To me, it didn't matter that he hadn't perforated anyone before. It didn't matter that these risks were rare. Rare means nothing to someone that has already experienced the trauma of rare. And I told him this. I had convinced myself that I would not see the other side of this procedure, that I would be a part of the statistics that made up the "risks." I gave my husband, "The Note" as they rolled me into my procedure, so that he could have some last words, and share them with our children, if anything were to happen.

I was wrong…

If catastrophic,
earth shattering,
devastating loss,
brought me to my faith?

What on earth
could ever pull me away?

I thought there was nothing.
I've already been dealt the very worst hand,
God-given pain,
of the very worst kind.

And I leaned in.
I leaned in.

I ran to,
and not away.
Leapt in,
and not out.

Wild horses could not drag me away.
Nothing could lead me astray.

I was wrong.
I was wrong.

In My Strength

I don't want to feel angry –
But I am.

I don't want my faith to be shaken –
But it is.

I don't want my trust to be broken –
But it appears that it has.

I want to believe that You have good plans for me –
But I don't.

I want to be able to run into Your arms –
But I can't.

I want to believe in the power of prayer –
But I'm not sure I do.

I want to believe in a loving God –
But where is He.

I want to draw near –
But I'm distancing.

I want to believe You are the same today,
as you were yesterday –
But I now see You as different.

I want to believe You are with me in the storm –
But I can't look past that You were the creator of it.

I want to get through this in Your strength –
But I now choose to do it in mine.

Thought you should know... I let the Lord lead me and I felt completely misled. For the first time since losing Mallory, I did not want the Lord to be the rock on which I stood. Every truth was in question. I praised Him in the valley and I just did not know how to praise Him through this. I couldn't comprehend how a loving God had led me to this place of complete surrender fully knowing what lie ahead. I did not want to get through in His strength anymore, but my own.

Don't Pray for Me

Please don't pray for me,
although I know that you mean well.

Look how much you already have,
yet the pieces…
still fell,
where they fell.

Our Lord,
our God has a plan,
despite the words we pray.

So please don't waste
your precious breath.
He will do it in His own way.

How many times
can the outcome be
exactly the opposite
of what we asked of He?

His will is His will,
and His plan is His plan,
and it really doesn't matter
all the requests of man.

Apparently
one day,
it will all make sense.

IF…
He sees fit to reveal it
when we're on His side of the fence.

And truly if
we make it there,
the full landscape and big picture,
I don't think we'll care.

The intricacies…
The details…
Will we really care to know?

Me?

I just want to be back with my people.
So I can live new…
and let go.

Thought you should know… Even prayer felt in question. An army of people had prayed for me while Mallory was in the hospital. A smaller army of people were praying for me with the news of my new pregnancy. Prayers for health first and foremost. Yet despite all of these prayers, two big outcomes, the exact opposite of what was prayed for. I felt like prayer didn't work. God already has His plan. His will is His will and He has already determined our days. So many people were praying for me after the loss of the miscarriage and this poem was my way of saying don't bother. These are not my true feelings on prayer, but they were my true angry feelings at the time this poem was written.

My Fight

I've praised You in the valley,
in the depths of despair.
I've trusted Your promises,
believed You to be there.

I believed You to be faithful,
loving and true.
I believed You to be just,
and to lead me on through.

How can You love me
when You've burdened me so?
How can I again trust You
to be all in the know?

You authored this story,
yet you're where I should run?
I ran straight to You last time.
But this time, I can't come.

I've lost relationships before.
Yet You, I can't lose.
But how do we grow without trust,
when I feel such doubt in Your truths.

Lord, I praised You in the valley.
I drank from Your fountain.
But what I longed for most
was to one day praise You on the mountain.

But I guess it was too much a request,
to take me on height.
So I will climb up alone.
This is mine now to fight.

The Target

Lord, how many storms
can one person take?
Why keep choosing the same target,
making the same person break?

My training in pain?
Is it still not complete?
Are you still anointing me for something greater,
by dishing out pain on repeat?

Is this pain for protection?
Avoidance of something down the road?
Will I see it when I get there?
That you were actually lightening my load?

What will you do next, Lord?
Who next will you take?
Why not just say what you want from me,
without making my entire world shake?

I'm constantly in your word.
I listen in prayer.
I don't understand your methods.
They feel cruel… and unfair.

Was I not obedient enough?
Did my praise fall far short?
I just have so many questions,
and through them I can't sort.

But I don't want You to sort them.
No. I don't want that from You.
I'm not seeking Your answers,
nor to be near to You.

You go that way,
and me, I'll go this…

And if truly Your faithful,

well then please Lord…
forgive me of this.

At Least

I can look back and say
that I did all that I could.
That I gave You all of me,
as I was encouraged I should.

My worries,
My fears…
All lifted to you.

The key
to that one compartment…
Trusted to You.

I won't have to look back
wondering what could have been,
thinking, "if only I had surrendered
way back when."

I bent to Your will.
I followed Your lead.
I trusted You as provider
to know what I'd need.

I'm proud of that woman,
who was terrified but let go.
What happened in the after
was not in her control.

But at least she doesn't have to wonder,
what her life could be,

if all those years ago
she would have submitted to He.

Because she did it.
It's done.
She gave herself to the One.

And He showed her.
He showed her.
He showed the outcome.

Thought you should know... This poem was my way of finding a "silver lining." It was my way of purposing the pain. I would never have to torture myself with the what ifs. I would never have to wonder what life would be like if I let go and let God. Because I did fully surrender. I did fully submit. And I knew the outcome. It wasn't the outcome I wanted but it was an outcome indeed. This poem was to honor my obedience.

Glorious Bow

I used to feel hope
with Your glorious bow.
The safety of Your promise
in the vibrant colors it shows.

But now that I look back,
on each and every time,
I see it as an omen –
a big warning sign.

A storm is a brewing,
and there's no place I can hide.
A storm is a brewing,
about to change the tide.

I don't know what it is,
and I don't know when it's coming,
But when I see that glorious rainbow,
I'll be sure to start running.

Thought you should know... I saw a rainbow outside my window right after Brian and I talked about trying for another baby. I saw a rainbow right after I got the news that we were having another girl. These rainbows did not feel like coincidence. They felt like confirmation. The Lord had his hands in this. After losing the pregnancy, rainbows had a different feel. I felt that I misinterpreted them.

The Valley

I am learning that new grief
heightens the grief already there.
That they instantly latch onto each other,
and strengthen as a pair.

They intertwine, intersect,
bind you into a hold.
They drain you of all progress
and turn everything cold.

They throw you back to the valley,
but this time it feels deeper.
You're lower than before,
and feel all the more weaker.

The sad part is, you don't even fight it.
You've been re-beaten, re-broken,
and there's just no way to right it.

There's no damn point in even trying to get out.
Just sit there and rot…
feel the hope seep out.

"You win," whoever's after me.
"Have it your way."

"I refuse to take one step.
In the valley,
I'll stay."

The Wheel

Give me back the wheel –
the one I gave over to You.

I'd rather be in the driver's seat,
even though I don't know what to do.

I'll set the route.
And any detours.

This way when I crash…

It's my fault.
and not Yours.

Postpartum or Grief

Is it postpartum or grief?
How could I know,
when the signs and the symptoms
so similarly show.

Sadness.
Hopelessness.
No thing that brings pleasure.

Poor concentration.
Irritability.
No energy to measure.

Postpartum or Grief?
Both possibly?
Can I include that within this,
when there's no baby to see?

You see, each and every other time,
there was a physical baby, that I could call mine.

But this time, there's no baby in hand.
Yet I feel all those old feelings
taking over my land.

Is this postpartum plus grief?
I fear that it is.
My baby's not here
but my body knows no difference.

Postpartum Anxiety

Is this postpartum? The anxiety kind?
Are you allowed to call it that,
when there's no baby to find?

You see, each and every other time,
there was a physical baby
that I could call mine.

The anxiety, the worry,
would overtake me,
with the immense responsibility
of a new baby.

But it wasn't my fault!
It was my body's way.
How it responded to hormones
going every which way.

But this time, there's no baby in hand.
Yet the familiar fears, have shaken my land.

I find I can't breathe,
that my breath can't stay pace.
The beat of my heart –
a palpitating race.

Is this postpartum?
It just may be.
Someone tell my body,
"There's NO baby."

Everyone, but you…

While I can't stop the bleed,
you're basking in the sun.

While I can hardly breathe,
your world's still whole and one.

And sometimes this is the hardest part –
the unobstructed view.

Bearing witness to how life goes on –
for everyone but you.

The smiles. The laughter.
The happy ever after…

Sometimes it's too much to see.

I'm happy for you.
Yes, I'm happy for you.

But when can I be happy for me?

Your Ways

"For My thoughts are not your thoughts.
Neither are My ways your ways."

Well that's most certainly clear.
Because I never would find goodness, and glory,
in taking away loved ones so dear.

Nor would pain ever be my go to,
inflicting it on the chosen
to bring about some breakthrough.

No!
I'd be more like the God who came as an equal.

Teaching. Rebuking.
Performing miracles for His people.

I'd answer questions.
Make very clear the real plan.

I'd never go silent
or have you wondering
where I am.

The One who walked the earth,
He's who I'd be!
The One who healed. Who wept.
Who faced temptation…
like me.

Why

There are no more whispers of why.
No more shouting it into the night sky.

Why?

Because there is no answer,
that could ever,
possibly,
satisfy.

Prayer

"Keep on praying, with thanksgiving."
Colossians 4:2.

Lord I was doing this.
Each and every time
I prayed to You.

Thank you God,
for this beating heart.
Thank you God,
for this brand new start.

1 Thessalonians 5:16.
"Pray continually.
Pray without ceasing."

Lord I was doing this.
I was praying all day.

Please give this baby health.
Please let this baby stay.

"Ask and it will be given."

"Seek, and you will find."

I did this oh Lord.
But the open door,
I can't find.

Well…

I guess that's not fully true.
You opened the door,
but then You closed it too.

And that's where I'm stuck.
That's where I'm reeling.
To take back an answered prayer
filled with all sorts of healing.

But then I stumbled,
upon James 4:3 –
"You ask with wrong motives,
so you did not receive."

And I sit here and wonder.
Are You talking to me?
Were my motives not right,
to want a baby?

And now I don't know
how to come to You and pray.
As maybe the desires of my flesh
give me the wrong words to say.

So I will strictly give thanks
for the good that I see.
And I will NOT wish for more
than what You wish for me.

Prayer Request

Jesus, I'm really not sure what comes next.
Or how I even feel about this prayer request.

But if I'm really Yours,
and You're really mine,
maybe You can answer
this one prayer in time.

My family's been broken.
We live in deep grief.
And from the moment life shattered,
we clung tight to belief.

Belief that Your life,
the truth…
and the way.

Belief in Your promise –
of a new world…
someday.

Belief in a time
when we're whole again.
Belief in a world
that knows no sin.

This place, in our midst
where we're desperate to go…
The order we'll go…
well only You know.

And see,
this request of mine,
(in your right time)
it has all to do
with our limits on time.

We've lived in deep grief!
Such hardship we've shared!

We can't do separation!

Some here.
And some there.

So take us at once.
Just come for us all.
Let us go together
when You come to call.

Hear me my Lord.
It's the only way.
Please take us together.
In Your name, I pray.

I'm Angry

I'm angry that I'm expected to carry on.
That I'm expected to stand back up
and walk across the broken glass…

AGAIN –
with grace.

I'm tired of sifting through the rubble.
I'm tired of putting the ashes through a sieve
to find any semblance of a future
that is salvageable.

There is nothing that feels salvageable.
Not when another key piece to the equation is missing.

I resent that I AGAIN have to create balance
out of a remainder.
That I have to use what's left of what's left
to form a new normal.

I HATE new normals.

And the worst part…

I'm expected to put my trust,
my faith,
my hope
into the One
who could've stopped this,
who AUTHORED this.

I'm supposed to believe
AGAIN
that this is for my good
and His glory.

How can someone say that to me
with a straight face?

I don't want to go to Him.

But where else do I go?
Who else do I look to?
What is my alternative?

The truth is…

I'm desperate for the hope.
I'm desperate for the promises.

For death not to have the final word.
For pain not to have the everlasting say.

So I guess I'll crawl along the broken glass.

Right back –
to the hand that struck me.

Another Chance

Perhaps I'm most angry at myself.

For letting my guard down.
For allowing myself to look ahead.
For falling in love with a tomorrow,
that was not yet my today.

I know better.
Yes…
I know better.

I allowed my imagination to get the best of me.

My feet –
to run ahead of me.

I set my eyes on
a new horizon.

My heart beat with renewed purpose –

The gift of life
and not just the sting of death.

The gift of life.

Thump-thump, thump-thump.

The gift of life…

Lord, Where Are You

Lord, where are You in this?
I search, yet cannot find.
I feel void of Your spirit,
leaving me to the vultures of my mind.

Lord, I have eyes, yet do not see.
I have ears, but do not hear.
I'm reaching out my hand,
but I find nothing of You near.

Lord, why have You left me?
How long will I stay alone?
Why keep me in this darkness?
Shine a light to bring me home.

Lord, am I even Yours?
Have You really chosen me?
I need something to believe this so.
I need a sign to blatantly see.

Or am I one that got away.
Never really in Your plan.
One the enemy would eventually enter.
An example, of the kind You ban.

Lord, show me where You are.
It's critical I see.
I need to know where I stand.
I need to know… that Your… with me.

Childlike Faith

How they must feel –
day out and day in,
when mommy doesn't want
to get out of bed again.

And while they don't understand –
where her mind's been,
they don't tug her out…
they gently climb in.

They crave her return –
but they don't demand when,
having faith in the timing,
trusting her…
to Him.

Thought you should know… This poem is inspired by my children. They had a front seat view of my emotional recovery of the pregnancy loss. Not once did they have comments or questions that showed their faith in question. Their childlike faith was beautiful to witness. Their complete trust in Him was a beautiful encouragement to me.

Both Matter

No one hesitates to congratulate.

Quick to praise.
Quick to applaud.
Quick to toast or
commend our good God.

Yes, there's no wait to congratulate.

But when things go south,
and there are no good words
to come out of the mouth…

We hesitate.
We procrastinate.

There's a lull and a lag.
We pause and we drag.

It's easier to congratulate than it is to commiserate.

But I'm here to say,
for both you shouldn't wait.
Not to offer condolences.
And not to congratulate..

BOTH matter.
BOTH carry weight.
Pay tribute to both.
Do not hesitate.

Linear

Grief is not linear.
And neither is one's walk with the Lord.

One step forward,
and two steps back.

A glimpse of the light,
before it all turns black.

Resting and wrestling.
Wrestling and resting.

Time filled with peace.
And time of real testing.

Grief is not linear
And faith is not too.

Yet grief without faith,
that is NOT the way through.

Wherever you stand, on either road.
He's walking with you,
He desires your load.

Letting Go

Everyone says
the hardest part is letting go.
But I, don't think so.

I let go.
And boy, was I scared.
But I should have held on.
I shouldn't have dared.

I let go,
and I lost.

And letting go
wasn't worth
what it cost.

And that's the hardest part, you see.
Living with the aftermath
of what broke within me.

The letting go was supposed to set free.

But instead –
it weighted down
what was already too heavy.

And now I go about
with more on my plate.
With more on my mind.
With a worsened state.

So I should have held on,
should have never let go.
I was better before.

Before, I let go.

Thought you should know... I wanted to take back my surrender. I had lost my two year old child and by God's grace had found some balance in my life. I teetered on the edge for so long – should I or shouldn't I – in trying for a new baby. I finally took the leap as an act of obedience, and now I wished I could take the leap back. The whole experience shook my world. There was no more balance. Everything felt heavier, my plate fuller. This poem is inspired by those very real feelings.

The Ride

"The ride was worth the fall."

I just can't say that here.
It doesn't feel that way.
At all.

What did I achieve?
What did I gain?

Only false hope.
Only more pain.

I can't justify the journey.
I can't rationalize the blow.

The experience NOT worth the setback.
The high NOT worth the low.

I wasn't looking to grow my family,
inside the heavenly plane.

I was looking to grow it here!
Inside the earthly domain.

The ride has given bitterness.
Left a sullen, sour taste.

The ride has damaged faithfulness,
transforming trust to convicted waste.

The ride was anything but worth it.
The value, I cannot find.

Yet God, doesn't waste a hurt.

But the cost…
it has made me blind.

Lord, I pray I one day see it.
That this ride was worth this fall.

Lord, I pray that You unveil it,
when Your kingdom comes to call.

The Waiting Room

I am the outsider in this place.
I no longer fit inside this space.

The walls feel like they're caving in,
as the expecting women
keep closing in.

All here, because they're on pace.
I'm afraid I'll scare them,
if they can read my face.

I can't make eye contact
or look their way.
I almost bolt for the door.
"I can't do this today."

My heart starts racing.
I can't catch my breath,
knowing they're here because of life,
and I'm here because of death.

And without meaning to,
I give one a quick glance.
She rests her hand on her belly,
and it sets me into a trance.

What if her appointment,
it goes like mine.
She's here all alone,
thinking everything's fine.

But what if her appointment,
shouts silence like mine.
What if her appointment
is like mine that last time.

And I hear myself whisper,
"No, please no…"
I tug these thoughts out of my head…
"Go, please go…"

But my wild expression,
sadly, gets the woman's attention.

"Are you alright?
You look kind of gray?"

"Me? Oh I'm fine.
Yea… I'm okay."

"I have crackers if you need."
She thinks it's nausea to blame.
I'm fumbling for words,
but saved by the sound of my name.

I get up to go in,
but I glance back her way.

"Good luck," I muster,
"with your appointment today."

The Shoes

It always felt
too good to be true.
Like I was squeezing my foot
into an old shoe.

Holding on
to what once was my style.
Forcing that fit
to walk a new mile.

But these treasured shoes,
once easily slipped on,
blistered my feet,
like they didn't belong.

I didn't want to acknowledge it.
I'd break them back in.
Like riding a bike,
or remembering to swim.

I desperately wanted
to fill those same shoes.

But life…
sometimes we win,
and sometimes we lose.

I've retired the shoes.
And all I hoped they would be.
I've retired the shoes, no longer meant for me.

A Mother's Instincts

We've never met
face to face.
But I know I'll know you
when I get to your place.

Don't ask me how.
It's just one of those things.
I'll pick you out of a crowd.
A mother's instincts.

And the beautiful thing
is you'll know me too.

You're here, Mommy.
I've been waiting for you.

Due Date

When a due date comes and goes.
And no one even knows…

Well, it's another kind of alone.
A pain, that's all your own.

You carried a life
that truly mattered.

Experienced a loss
that left you shattered.

But because the world didn't get to hold them.

Love them.
Meet them.
Know them.

It feels their gone
without a trace.
Yet in your heart,
they hold a space.

And even though you didn't get to meet them.

Hold them.
Love them.
Greet them.

For you…

The due date won't come
and go.

You'll remember.
Always,
you'll know.

Thought you should know… The first thing anyone asks when they find out you're pregnant. "When are you due?" December 19th 2025. That's when I was due. I know in my heart that day is going to come and go and no one will remember. I will remember. I'll always remember.

Dear Lord

I have forgotten how to pray. My mind comes to You, I think of You, all throughout my day. But when it comes time to kneel and pray, I do not have the words to say. I hold unforgiveness in my heart. And I know that's not Your way. But I cannot seem to speak it out when I come to You to pray.

Maybe it's because when I speak it, I may be expected to release it. But I still want to hold to it tight. I feel like I have every right. But I know that is not true. Forgiveness is a core principle, as a follower of You.

Lord, the unforgiveness in my heart, I know that you well know. I hold it all towards You, for a way You did not show. And in my unwillingness to let it go, this unforgiveness, it has dared to grow. I don't know how to talk to You about it. I haven't prayed because I'm incapable of talking around it.

To start the conversation, would be the beginning of working it through. But I just can't seem to get there. I can't bring myself to You.

Lord, when you forgive, you do so completely. You blot out our wrongdoings, and You do so repeatedly. The bible says, "You forgive our transgressions as far as the east from the west." You do so abundantly, giving our minds this blessed rest.

How come I can't do it back, Lord? Forgive you, like you do me? Maybe it's because there's nothing to forgive. And it has to be me with the apology. I'm told you don't make mistakes, Lord. That you have an all-knowing and perfect plan. And I'm not meant to understand it… as I'm not God, but man.

And so I'm left in the same situation, at a total loss of what I should pray. Because I think You owe me an apology, for all the pain You've repeated my way. But I know I have it all wrong Lord. The offence, it can't be on You. I'm singing all the wrong chords, Lord. I've lost… the beat… of Your truth.

I'll make this my one prayer Lord. Forgive me what I just can't let go. Because even amidst unforgiveness, You're where I'm still longing to go.

Griever

Barren Land

What to do when the rock on which I stand,
now feels like barren land.

Others keep planting seeds.
But what grows is unfruitful.
What grows is just weeds.

All they can do is pray and plant.
But it's Him who can answer.
It's Him who can grant.

All they can do is water and sow.
But it's Him who can bloom.
It's He who makes grow.

Have I become sterile ground?
Have I become an infertile mound?

What once bore fruit,
now desolate and bleak.

That once strong root,
now struggling and weak.

My Lord. My God.

Tend to this garden.
Soften this soil.
Unstiffen what's hardened.

My Lord. My God.

Water this hole.
Nourish what's Yours.
Save this lost soul.

You'll do it my Lord.
You'll do it.
You must.

You'll do it, dear God.
You'll do it.
I trust.

New Believer – A Variation

I had this insatiable appetite.
Hungered –
for no one but You.
A beggar for more of Your word, God.
Like I'd been starved
before I'd met You.

Your words satisfied my cravings.
They nourished my soul needing saving.

Their richness made me alive.
I was no longer failure to thrive.

Your word,
like the milk of a mother.
It's fullness –
grew me,
like no other.

Available right on demand.
A force in the palm of my hand.

It knew exactly what I needed.
Power in each and every feeding.

I became a new creation.
as the fruitfulness coursed on through,
The old me passed away,
and I was born again, made new.

Then Lord, something happened.
You didn't show up, as I'd imagined.

My appetite became less and less.
My trust turned into unrest.

And now again, I'm failing to thrive.
I've been force-feeding Your word,
just trying to survive.

Yet daily when I reach for Your bread.
I choke on what once
brought me back
from the dead.

Help me, oh Lord.
My hardness has taken a toll.
Help me, oh God,
Feed this weathered, cold soul.

Hold onto me Heaven

Hold onto me Heaven.

I'm straining
maintaining
my grip.

Hold onto me Heaven.

I'm terrified
any second
I'll slip.

Hold onto me Heaven.

I'm being pulled
toward a blackened abyss.

Can't you see I'm under attack Heaven?

I need you
to help me
with this.

I'm just barely hanging on.

Wrestling.
Writhing.
Being lured for too long.

Hold onto me Heaven.
Don't let me go wrong.

Hold onto me Heaven.
My might almost gone.

Hold onto me Heaven.
Please help me stay strong.

Hold onto me Heaven.
The home I so long.

Hold onto me Heaven.
To you… I belong.

Hold onto me Heaven.
I'm singing your song.

Hold onto me Heaven.
Your light be shone.

Hold onto me Heaven.
Darkness… be gone.

The Word of the Lord

I wrestle with it,
all the while,
I rest within it.

It's like how can this be true,
all the while,
I just need it to.

So I grapple,
while I grasp.

I battle,
while I clasp.

I struggle,
while I grip.

I hold tighter,
while I slip.

Because Your Word, it is the way.
And from it, I will not stray.

Please forgive me,
all my wrestling.
Please empower me,
in all this testing.

Because in You, I'm still resting.
Yes, in You, I'm still resting.

Your Armor

Let us hold on
to the confession of our hope
without wavering,
since he who promised is faithful.
(Hebrews 10:23)

Lord, help me.
I hold on to the hope like a lifeline.

But I waver.

I waver in my testing.
I waver in my suffering.

I am most viciously attacked
when lost in this wilderness of affliction,
when adrift in this sea of vulnerability.

And the lies…

They seep into my heart.
They bleed into my brain.

And they probe
and poke holes
in Your believability.

The questions start swirling.
Questions that all start like this:

How can a good God...

And I start living,
in a bed, of mistrust.

I ink question marks,
all over Your word.

I cast shadows,
all over Your plan.

I throw shade at my very own salvation.

I harp on the scriptures that come with real warning:

They always go astray in their hearts,
and they have not known my ways.
So I swore in my anger,
they will not enter my rest.
(Psalm 95:10-11)

And I fear You are speaking to me.

How many times can my heart go astray
before you harden like this against me?

How many times can I crawl back Your way
before I no longer get respite in thee?

Lord, my soul seeks Your rest.
But I slip further away
with each and every test.

Help me to stand in the strength of Your Armor.

Put Your truth like a belt on my waist.
Your righteousness like armor on my chest.
Your peace like sandals on my feet.
So that in every situation,
I can extinguish all the flaming arrows
of the evil one.
(Ephesians 6:14-16)

Whispers

The devil comes whispering in my ear,
breathing life into every fear.

He constantly tells me I'm no good,
that I definitely can't do
what I think I may should.

But each and every single time,
he disguises himself
as if a friend of mine.

And I follow his lead.
Believe every word.
Measure myself
against his lies I've been told.

The shame seeps in.
The anger, regret.
And I see myself
as someone I'd like to forget.

My world gets darker.
My hope bleeds out.
My circle gets smaller,
and I just see no way out.

But without fail,
as I reach my ropes end,
I come face to face
with my savior again.

He gently lifts
me off the ground,
despite the filth
in which I've been found.

No disgracing.
No scolding.
No "again, you've gone astray."

Just arms wide open
to come back
His way.

Angel Sisters

Two sisters –
joined in my heart.
Introduced after death –
did us all part.

One handpicked
by the other.
But not for the pleasure
of their earthly mother.

One handpicked
to directly be flown,
to her angel sister
in her heavenly home.

Together they wait,
in perfect form,
as the most beautiful rainbow
after this earthly storm.

What a glorious reunion
I know it will be,
when these two angel sisters
are rejoined… with me.

Safe and Secure

The pardon the interruption is over.
There's nothing more to convey.

But I will never forget the season,
a dream shone, then darkened away.

It's not that I'm better or over it.
It's that there's nothing more to say.

And for the benefit of me, my family,
I had to step into the light of new day.

I had to tuck this loss,
and all it came with,
securely and safely away.

Section II – Concluding Thoughts

Please know how difficult it was to share much of the poetry in this section. I have painstakingly gone over it again and again and again, the questions are always the same. Should I take this one out? Is it okay to say that? Will I come off as not a true follower? Am I dishonoring the Lord with my angry words? Dishonoring Him is something that I would never want to do.

My immediate response after the loss of Mallory was to run to the Father, arms I had never run into before. I stood on His word and a platform of hope and love. I professed my belief and testimony in public forums. I chose baptism on what would have been Mallory's 3rd birthday as an outward expression of my faith. Brian and I renewed our vows on this same day, exchanging promises that put the Lord in our marriage. We felt we didn't do this the first time around and wanted to right that wrong. Neither one of us wanted to live life anymore without God in it, including our marriage. Especially our marriage.

I say all this because even in my anger, I cannot and will not deny what the Lord has done for me. And He did something for me in the aftermath of the miscarriage, too. He led me to my journals. He led me back to my very first journal entries in the days and weeks following the loss of Mallory. I reread ALL of them. And I was reminded that on October 1, 2023, just ONE day after burying my child, I went to my very first church service.

A lightbulb went off in my head as I remembered what that sermon was about. *Deconstruction of Faith.* It meant nothing to me at the time really because I wasn't deconstructing, I was being pulled to belief for the first time. I was *constructing.* But I was at this difficult crossroads right now. The Lord led me to my journals. He reminded me of this sermon. Perhaps He was telling me to go back and watch it. So I did.

And wow. It blew my mind that the Lord planted a sermon in my path 2 years before I would need its message. It blew my mind that He lovingly led me back to this sermon through the gift He had given me – written expression. If I had not journaled, I would not have remembered this sermon. Here is what I think He wanted me to understand.

The pastor defined deconstruction as an undoing of one's accepted beliefs about God. He explained that deconstructions usually come about because God did not provide in a way that one thought He would, like He went off script, leaving you questioning if God can really be who you thought He was.

Well that was me right there. God did not provide in this circumstance as I thought He would. It did feel like He went off script. I was questioning if He was who I thought He was.

But the pastor said this… "Just because you have questions and doubts, it does not mean you need to walk away. Maybe this deconstruction project is necessary to put your faith back together stronger than before."

He then turned to the church community. He said let us not be a place where questions and questioners are not welcome. He said let us listen first. Then let us be a real person and share our struggles back, share that we too at some point have wrestled. He gave examples of prominent people who wrestled with God in the bible. Jacob. David. Moses. Abraham. The Psalmists. Even Jesus wrestled. And then he said exactly what I needed to hear. He said exactly the words that I feel the Lord led me back to this sermon to rest in. He said, "If you are wrestling with your faith, that is the surest sign that you actually have one." What a comfort those words were to me!

Being led back to this sermon was the first sign of feeling the Lord with me in this circumstance. He was telling me that my questions and doubts are okay, normal even. He was reminding me that my wrestling, and my writing, was actually my way of pursuing Him, my way of staying connected.

This sermon allowed me to rest in my decision to keep all the angry and unfiltered lament-like poetry within this book. I took nothing out, watered nothing down. It is important to me to be a place where questions and questioners feel welcome. I want to listen, and be a real person, and share back, "I've been there too. And it's okay."

And then I will ask them the same question that I had to ask myself. Is turning away a better option? For me, the answer is no.

Section III

For me, the answer is no. There is ONE thing that holds more weight than any of the other emotions in grief combined.

HOPE. One little glimmer of hope lights up my entire darkened world. And that is the hope of Heaven.

I believe that my daughter lives in Heaven, that Jesus welcomed her into His loving arms. I believe He wiped every tear from her eye. I believe she is free from the pain and suffering that her earthly body came to know in her final days, and that she lives in a place that is eternally free of all those things. I believe this wholeheartedly, even though I did nothing to teach her about Jesus while she was here. I believe this because Jesus tells us this. "Let the little children come to me," He says, "and do not hinder them, for the kingdom of heaven belongs to such as these." Matthew 19:14.

HOPE. Tell me… where else can I find it except through Him? Where else is there a promise like this one, except through Him? There has got to be more than the sufferings of this world, and He promises there is.

People always say, "I don't know how you do it," as if I have some sort of superhuman strength. I can assure you that I have no such strength. This is how I do it. I cling to the hope of Heaven. I cling to the hope that I too, will have every tear wiped from my eye. I too, will be freed from the pain and suffering my earthly body has come to know. And that I will live free… and forever united with my child… my children, in a home that He provides us. However shaken, and while so much does not make sense, it's a hope I will not walk away from.

The Reason

My first time in deep grief,
no one actually died.
In fact, who I was grieving,
was very much alive.

But I learned that this person…
wasn't who I thought,
that the gestures he showed me,
were premediated… well thought.

He was grooming,
and primping,
and claiming to be…

Someone he wasn't –
and he completely fooled me.

But I was only a child.
How could I know?
That his love,
and affection,
were all just a show.

A big demonstration,
a performance,
an act…

I trusted his expression.
Took him for fact.

And after it all,
came to bright light,
he was just gone from my life –
banished from sight.

And all the love I still had,
I had to hide it away.
Because I knew it wasn't acceptable
to still feel that way.

All who adored him,
filled with such hate.
And I knew it was expected,
I reciprocate.

And so outwardly, I did.
All day I would hate.
While inwardly I hid,
my devastation so great.

But now I'm an adult,
And I won't hide anymore.
I loved you, now hate you
for my innocence you tore.

You are the reason,
I needed control.
You are the reason,
I was never quite whole.

You are the reason,
I carried such doubt,

that I questioned my worth,
that my voice couldn't shout.

You are the reason,
I mistrusted people so.
You are the reason,
I couldn't go with the flow.

You are the reason,
I held on too tight.
You are the reason
I'd let go with no fight.

You are the reason,
I was afraid of unknowns.
You are the reason,
I'd take thrown stones.

You are the reason,
I was fearful of change.

Because that day changed
EVERYTHING –
my whole life rearranged.

But… you are the reason,
I built me a dream.

There was a world I wanted back,
a life to redeem.

You are the reason,
for the paths that I chose.
the terrain that I've journeyed,
big climbs and deep lows.

And I realize now
with crystal clear eyes,
that a lifetime of behavior
was this deep grief in disguise.

And today is the day,
I take back your power.
You WERE the big reason.
but GONE is your hour.

Thought you should know... I learned early on that a single curve can change the trajectory of your life forever. This poem was to process a defining experience during my formative years. It took the loss of my daughter, and all the feelings it came with, to understand that a lifetime of behavior was rooted in a grief of a different kind. I allowed that experience to put a hold on me. To shape me. This poem gives voice to that pain and release to the trauma that I was not ready to let go of.

The World Keeps Dancing

How is it the world keeps dancing?
It doesn't skip a beat!
It taps on like nothing happened.
Pirouettes on pointed feet.

It twirls in perfect balance.
Plié's amidst the storm!
It goes from varying positions,
with fluid and perfect form.

How is it the world keeps dancing?
Hoes does it not even skip a beat?
It just continues on performing!
The same old dance… just on repeat.

Doesn't it hear the music's stopped?
Doesn't it sense the world's gone wrong?
Isn't there anything that can halt it?

Must the show
ALWAYS
go on!

Yes the world just keeps on dancing.
And to me –
that's the hardest part.

What they see as graceful movements,
feels like harsh stomping on my heart.

Yes the world just keeps on dancing.
But to me,
the music's died.

I no longer feel the beat,
of the world's rhythm,
I once relied.

I am no dancer in the street,
since the day
my person
died.

Death Came

Death came,
like a thief in the night.
It stole memories.
And milestones.
And a future so bright.

Death pounced in,
like a predator to prey.
A ruthless ambush
in the light of day.

Death wreaked havoc,
like a hurricane to shore.
A storm surge to the mind,
and a foundation no more.

Death spun in,
like a tornado touching ground,
uprooting life as I'd known it,
leaving nothing as it found.

Death lingered,
like a fog in the air,
leaving no compass needle
to the wilderness out there.

Death darkened,
like an eclipse of the sun,
obscuring the view
and demanding attention.

Death struck,
invading my space,
leaving behind a cold sting
from a sharp slap in the face.

Death imposed,
like an unwanted guest.
forcing its will,
and disrupting what's best.

Yes death waged war.
A most vicious attack.
It demolished a world,
we can never get back.

Death drew,
a line in the sand,
creating a before and an after,
and no choice where you stand.

But death has lost.
The battle's been won.
The sting, not permanent.
Praise be… to the Son.

I suspect…

I have this sneaking suspicion,
that despite time's great ambition…

The worst year of grief,
may always just be,
the one
in which
I am living.

The Current

Grief is an unpredictable current
of calm waters
and raging seas.

Do not try to swim against it.

Flow with it.
Float when you can.

Tread.

Ride the waves.
And hold on.

Always, hold on.

Buried

I stood at your casket,
as they dropped it down.
Lower and lower,
into the loose ground.

Flower after flower –
tossed on top.
Tears upon tears –
could not be stopped.

But it wasn't just you,
covered up that day.
It wasn't just you,
buried away.

I may still walk this solid ground.
And I can still be… physically found.

But something died in me that day.
And they buried it with you,
in that site where you lay.

Yes something died in me that day.

And they buried it with you.
In that place.
Where you lay.

Dying

Dying –
gradually ceasing to exist or function;
in decline and about to disappear.

That's how the dictionary defines it.

And that's what happened.
That's what I witnessed.

You –
dying.

You –
gradually ceasing to function.

You –
in decline,
and about to disappear.

But the dictionary doesn't have it all right.
No, it has some things so very wrong.

You did not cease to exist, my love.

Your body, yes.
But your soul, no.

I feel you still out there.
And I know where you are.

You see…
death means life for a believer.

You didn't decline and disappear.

Rather…
You journeyed a passageway to home.

Ecclesiastes 12:7
And the dust
returns to the earth
as it once was,
and the spirit
returns to God,
who gave it.

Dying – not gradually ceasing to exist.

But slowly… beginning… to live.

Funerals

I've been to many funerals.
I've waited on the line.
I've exchanged personal stories –
the once upon a times.

I've sent a floral arrangement.
I've dressed in all black.
I've perused all the pictures,
lining the tables in the back.

I've expressed my condolences.
I've kneeled down in prayer.
I've wrapped my arms around the family.
Looked into their teary, weary stare.

I've listened to the eulogies.
And the Pastor's threads of light.
I've followed the funeral processional,
stood at the final resting site.

Yes, I've been to many funerals.
Too many in my time.
But nothing could prepare me,
for when the family struck…
was mine.

The notes on the flowers –
all written out to me.

The pictures on the table –
of me, my family.

All the personal stories,
and the "waiters" on the line –
Celebrating a life
of a person that was mine.

To be the receiver of the sorry's,
and the voice behind the speech,
it's an inexplicable feeling,
no previous funeral can teach.

Sitting the front row.
Being the first car behind that hearse.
Forever, I've been changed.
Truly… nothing worse.

Thought you should know… No one can prepare you for an experience like this. This poem is to pay tribute to anyone who knows what it feels like to be the family that is center stage at a funeral.

Year 1

The year of the numbness.

You know what has happened,
but you move through the world in this slow
and surreal sort of way.

You know you are sad.
You know you are broken.

You know life as you knew it has ended
and that every single thing,
big or small,
has changed.

But you do not fully feel it.

You take each breath,
each moment,
each day,
each first,
as it comes.

Because what else can you do,
except merely exist,
in this world that just keeps on turning.

Magical Doorway

There must be some magical doorway
that grievers pass through on their own timeline.

For some it's instantaneous.
While for others, it's quite delayed.
But you'll know when you've reached it.

Because as soon as you enter…

The numbing enchantments wash off.
The film over your eyes lifts.
The guards surrounding your heart and mind disperse.

And you can see.
And you can feel.

Fully.

For the first time.

The true landscape of the wreckage takes shape.
The faded colors of this new world, exposed.

The magnitude of the loss,
plus the permanency of the pain –
"big bang" a new universe.

A new cosmological model established on one key principle:

"They are gone. And they are not coming back."

Shock re-enters like an intruder.
It choke-holds any forward progress.
It tramples on any sort of growth.

Their light,
that shone within you,
overshadowed
by complex emotions.

Sadness has stopped showing itself with tears.
Anger has infiltrated the mind.
Envy has entered the eyes.
Bitterness has broken into the heart.
Loneliness has crept inside the soul.

And joy… joy is nowhere to be found.

These invaders cannot be escaped,
even amongst your own handpicked crowd,
even within the net of your own safety.

And it all just feels too heavy.
It all just feels too much.

And to pile on to the too much,
the rest of the world enters their own magical doorway.
One that tells them you should be doing better.

You'll know they've entered when…

The check-ins lessen.
The empathy wanes.

The army retreats.

You find yourself battling the lonely… alone.

And you can't help but wonder.
Is this just life now?
Are there anymore magical doorways?
And if so, what will they bring?

You admittedly pray that you'll find one.

One that brings back the super natural numbing.
One that reestablishes the charmed film to the eyes.

And the guards…
Oh how you hope for those guards back.

May they stand watch again and forevermore.

Shielding the heart.
Protecting the mind.
Keeping the peace that passes all understanding.

May they shine a light in this blackened abyss.
So joy will peek her head out.
So she will settle down and stay
at least for awhile.

Never the Same

The loss of you,
continues to break me
in ways I cannot explain.

Even in days of sunshine,
I can't escape
the rain.

Yes, I move with it.
But each and every step,
not absent
of pain.

Yes, I go on.
But NEVER
the same.

NEVER –
the same.

Gravitational Pull

Sometimes I wonder if you truly knew,
how my whole wide world revolved around you.

What you wanted. What you needed.

Every day the same, our cycle repeated.

My whole wide world, revolved around you.
The gift of a lifetime, to orbit round you.

But now you're gone.
And I'm lost in space.
No gravitational pull,
in this vast, dark place.

Gone are the seasons.
Gone are the days.
Gone are the patterns
that purposed my ways.

How to touch ground
with no force of your pull.
A constant state of falling,
in this world with no you.

No sense of direction.
No up and no down.
Stuck in this medium,
with you not around.

Where You Left Off

You can't just pick up where you left off…
like others can.

You can't just close the door on the funeral
and open the door to a new day…
like others can.

Because for you,
each day brings a new funeral.

For you, each day, the same loss.

The Road Grows Quiet

In the beginning,
everyone jumps into the pit with you.

And when I say everyone,
I mean EVERYONE.

Friends.
Family.
Colleagues.
Acquaintances.
Neighbors.
Strangers.

People show up from near and they show up from far.

Card after card,
package after package,
meal after meal –
from people you know,
and from people you never met,
show up on your doorstep.

Every phase of your life
combines
and stands together
in solidarity
as you remember your person.

It's really quite something.

Truly –
quite something.

But the road grows quiet for the griever…
So very quiet.

Silence Speaks

So many go silent on us in our grief.

I'd be lying if I said it didn't hurt.
I'd be lying if I said it didn't confuse me,
or anger me, or make me wonder why.

"They don't know what to say," or
"They don't want to say the wrong thing."
That's the explanation I get from the ones who sit with me.
And I'm sure they're right.

But the truth is…

I'd rather them say SOMETHING over NOTHING.
I'd rather them say the WRONG thing over NO thing.

How about they just say I love you.
How about they just say I'm thinking of you.
How about they just say I don't know what to say,
but I want to be here for you.

How about they say her name.
Yes, her name.
How about they just say that.

Because silence speaks too ya know.
Yes. Silence speaks too.

It can even put words into your mouth.

Words like, "I don't love you."
Words like, "You never cross my mind."
Words like, "I have forgotten."

I don't know about you,
but I'd much rather say the wrong words with the best of intentions
than put out an unintended message spoken through silence.

But to each their own.
To each their own.

Changed

They say I've changed,
that I'm not who I used to be.

They're not wrong.
I am different.

But tell me…

What would they say about me
if I didn't change?

If I saw what I saw,
went through what I did,
and came out the same?

Change, or no change…
They'd be talking.

They haven't changed.

And maybe there lies the real problem.

Forgiveness

I do not have a desire to hear from these people again.

The people that showed up on that fateful day,
but did not show up again.

The people that watched me bury my child,
but have not sat with me since.

The people that listened to my eulogy
but have tuned me out thereafter.

No, I do not have a desire to hear from these people again.

But I do desire a peace with this secondary loss.

I desire to be liberated from the space
they take up in my mind,
the space they live "rent free"
inside my head.

I do not want an apology.
But, I do want to find a way to forgive.

Not so I can continue a relationship.
But so I can lift this extra
and unnecessary weight.

Forgiveness does not mean
we have to move on together.

It means letting go with no grudge.
It means releasing with no bitterness.
It means removing the chip off my shoulder.

The forgiveness is for you, yes.

But it's for me too.
It's for me too.

Thought you should know… I see forgiveness differently since my loss. I used to think forgiveness was more for the other person than it was for me. It is still that, yes! But forgiveness is so much for us too. When we don't forgive, we are harboring bitterness. We are making our daily load heavier. True forgiveness frees up this space in our heads. It warms the cold places in our heart. Being able to forgive is a grace for others AND it is a grace to ourselves.

Showing Up

Showing up means being present.

Some define present as being in a particular place.

But not me.
I don't define it that way.

I don't need you physically here to be present for me.

And I don't need to be physically where you are,
to be present for you.

The truth is,
one can be physically here,
but not really "here" at all.

To me,
present means showing up in one's circumstance.

It means "being there."

Not in body,
but in mind.

Not in a particular place –

But in words.
And in action.
And in spirit.
And in prayer.

Showing up –

It means everything.
Literally, EVERYTHING, to the griever.

I'll never forget who showed up for me.

And even more,

I won't forget who shows up still –
who shows up still.

Thought you should know… Many will show up for us in our grief. And the hard truth is, that many won't. Sometimes who you wouldn't expect to show up does, and who you would expect to show up doesn't. Our expectations of people and the roles they played in our lives prior to our loss are directly linked to how we think a person should or will show. What we expect and what actually happens do not always align.

Boundaries

Shutting people out
is not necessarily a bad thing
for a griever.

Maybe you are listening to your instincts.
Maybe it's a line in the sand long overdue.

Loss has a way of shifting things into perspective –

weeding out what needs to be weeded,
rooting down what needs to be planted.

Turning away from what no longer suits you
is a sign of healthy growth.

Yet others may see it
as a horn that needs to be blared,
or a red flag that needs to be raised.

Please don't allow those signaling
to blur those lines you created.

That boundary was set for a reason.

And those up in arms about it
are probably for whom it was drawn.

Please

Please,
with all due respect,
don't complain about your children in front of me.

Please don't share how tired you are.
Or how nutty they've been.
Or how stir crazy they are.

Please don't tell me how you just need a break,
or a little time to yourself.

Everything you are feeling is normal.
Yes, everything you are feeling IS normal.

But please don't tell it to me.

Because I'd take your reality,
over my reality,
any day.

Attention

I do not share my loss for attention.
I don't share it for likes…
or a mention.

I share for a person who mattered.
To honor a loss that left my heart shattered.

I share to keep my person known.
So her name is spoken beyond my home.

I share from a place of a love so deep.
A most precious person, I could not keep.

The Tortoise and the Hare

Grief, I'll let you set the pace.
I won't try to outrun.
There's no tortoise and hare.
This is no race to be won.

You fix the beat,
or change up the tone.

It doesn't need to be resolute.
Unbending.
In stone.

There's no conventional method.
No prearranged rules.
There's no customary standard.
Or pre-sharpened tools.

This is no road that's been fixed.
Or path that's been paved.

Yes, it's been traveled.
One MANY have braved.

But this road is our own,
and you set the pace.

Speed up or slow down
through the hurdles we'll face.

You fix the beat.
You change the tone.
I move to your rhythm.
And I sing to your groan.

You, not the tortoise.
And I, not the hare.

We journey together.

TOGETHER.
Out there.

Grieve – A Definition

Grieve –

To feel or express great sadness.

I've perused various definitions.

None of them directly state
to feel or express great sadness
BECAUSE
of the death of a loved one.

The majority of them say,
ESPECIALLY when it comes to the death of a loved one.

But still.

The definition leaves the word open to interpretation.

I've heard people use the word grieve
when talking about an estranged relationship.

I've heard people use the word grieve
with the loss of a job, or a home, or a move.

I've heard people use the word grieve
when talking about results of political elections.

I've heard people use the word grieve
when their children grow and leave the nest.

And I guess according to the dictionary definition,
they are technically not wrong.

Grieve does mean "to feel or express great sadness."

But I'd be lying if I said I didn't struggle with this.

Never have I seen a grief support group filled with empty nesters.
Or tied together because of an estrangement,
or a move, or a job.

Never have I seen grief serve a 4 year term.

Can we have very strong feelings on these things?

We sure can.
And we do!
We do.

But to grieve them…

Gratitude and Grief

I can be grateful for the time I had
AND grieve the time I lost.

I can be grateful for the memories I made
AND grieve all the memories I'll miss.

I can be grateful for the milestones reached
AND grieve the ones that never will be.

I can be grateful for the people I have
AND grieve those who've gone on.

It's not gratitude OR grief.

Its gratitude AND grief.

BOTH!

I can thank the Lord for the gifts He gives
AND question what He takes back.

I can trust God's promises
AND not understand what He's doing.

I can walk with Him.
AND I can wrestle.

BOTH!

Grief. Faith. Gratitude.

These are not one or the other.
They are not this way or that.

They are one AND the other.
They are this way AND that.

"What am I supposed to learn from this…"

Over and over,
again and again,
I hear this from different grievers.

I've even asked myself this question,
toyed with varying answers…

And truly it breaks my heart.

At times,
it even makes me MAD.

Too many grievers think that what happened to us
happened to us
because of us.

That there is a lesson
hidden
for us to uncover.

We do not need to learn some lesson from our loss.
WE DON'T!

Thinking that we do feels similar to saying
"There's a silver lining."

There is no silver lining!

Inadvertently, we do learn some things though, don't we.

We learn who our people are.
We learn the fragility of time.
We learn to take nothing for granted.
We learn how quickly life can change.
We learn how to cling onto little glimmers of hope.
We learn what matters and what doesn't.
We learn what we have room for and what we don't.
We learn our lack of control over life's curveballs.

Yes we learn so many things.

We learn there has to be more to life than this earthly realm.
There just has to be.

But not for one second am I telling you
that any one of these things,
is the silver lining.

There is no silver lining…
no silver lining.

What is God trying to develop through me?

I've pondered this.
Picked it apart.

Again and again,
I've asked Him.

God, what are you trying to develop through me?

And all that I can come up with is that I'm so sorry.

I'm sorry that I wasn't developed enough.
Or properly.
Or that I somehow grew wrong.

I grew so wrong that you had no choice
but to flood my world,
wipe it out.

All so I could reset.
All so you could develop something through me.

I'm sorry Lord that You had to do this.
I'm sorry there was no other way.

I'm sorry that I still don't know what it is
that You're trying to develop.

Now. Then. Always.

"I know it doesn't feel this way right now,
but it won't always be this hard.
I promise you, it will get easier."

This is what they tell me.
And this, in turn,
is what I hear.

That one day the heaviness of my loss will feel light.
That the grief in my heart won't always burn this bright.
That the grip constricting my airways won't stay this tight.

Essentially,
they are telling me,
time heals.

That it's okay for me to feel this way right now,
but at some point,
down the road,
later…

It will get better.

Let me be clear.
It will not get better.

A loss of this kind does not get easier.
Time will not heal it.

I know it's hard for you to understand this permanency.

But at some point,
down the road,
later…

Maybe you'll get it.

Stop setting a bar I won't reach.
Listen to what I'm trying to teach.

It will always be this heavy.
The grief is not temporary.
Actually, quite the contrary.

The grief doesn't lighten.
It will in fact brighten.
The chest remains tightened.

I broke on that fateful day.
I am broken, still, today.
And I will stay broken, the rest of the way.

I am grieving.

Now.
Then.
Always.

Grief Visual

I've seen many grief visual representations.

And there's some truth
to these illustrations.

Often shown,
is this big grief mass,
that keeps to its' size over time.

And the only thing that changes,
is how we grow around it with time.

We start off as a small little circle.
And the grief blob matches our size.

But we grow bigger around that grief blob.
Our proportions surpass its' bulked size.

And here's my synopsis on this.

I feel it's an errored depiction.
While I agree that we can grow around it,
let me paint you a different description.

The size of the mass
does NOT stay the same.
It can actually grow bigger
than the mass that first came.

As the days, months,
and the years pass on.
We lose them in more ways
than when they first were gone.

Memories and milestones
they never could know.
And as each one passes,
that grief blob grows.

We are constantly finding
new layers to grief,
so this illusion that it stays the same…
it is a false belief.

I can appreciate what the artist
is trying to do.
To drive home grief doesn't lessen
because that part is true.

But to claim that it stays
this same-sized ball.
Well that's just not true.
It's not true at all.

And another thing…

We as grievers,
we don't continually grow.
Grief is not linear.
And often backwards we go.

So as the days,
the months,
and the years pass on…

This narrative that we keep growing,
it's just plain wrong.

I'm not sure you can paint
an accurate image of grief.

It's just too damn individual.
To each it's unique.

"What are you up to today?"

It's a pretty harmless question.
For most.

But it isn't harmless for me.

You see,
it's a reminder.

A reminder of how my days used to be full.
How my time used to be spent.
How it was routined,
purposed,
planned out.

How every minute was centered on you.

Now my days feel empty.
Filled with longing,
and silence,
and ache.

Each day a blank slate.
I can fill the time as I choose.

But I still want to fill it with you.
I choose still… to fill it with you.

Open Wound

The loss of you will always be an open wound.
It's not that I'm grieving you still.
It's that I will grieve you always.

I will grieve you,
ALWAYS.

The Pain

There's nothing I've done to numb the pain.
Nothing.

You had no choice to feel what you lived through.
So why should I?

I try to imagine it sometimes.
What it must've been like for you.
To just want to feel better,
and looking to those you trusted most to make it so.

It makes me absolutely sick to my stomach.
SICK to my stomach.

But I don't do anything to ease it.
You couldn't ease it.
So why should I?

I'll feel every bit it.
Just like you did.

Small Talk

Polite conversation
about unimportant
or uncontroversial matters.

I can't do it in grief.

Talk to me real.
Or sit with me in silence.

But the small talk…
I can't do it.

I just can't do it in grief.

"One door closes and another door opens."

Not
in
grief.

Unless of course,

it's the door from one realm
to the other.

“This too shall pass.”

NOPE!

-or-

“This too shall pass.”

Yes!

When reunited.

Dear Support System

You must know that we grievers see your efforts.

We see your messages –
even if we don't respond.

We see your missed calls –
even though we don't always call back.

We appreciate your care package –
even though we don't always remember to say thank you.

We are grateful for your meal offer –
even though we don't always accept it.

We are thankful for your willingness to run an errand,
to do something hard alongside us,
to take the kids…
or whatever else it may be –
even though we still choose to do it ourselves and alone.

We know how you ache to listen –
even though we choose not to talk.

You must know that we see you, and that we love you –
even though we don't always show or express it.

And we thank you –
for being a constant in the chaos,
for being the beauty in the brutal,
for all of it.

We know we don't make it easy.

With love,
The Grievers

Flesh Angel

What about the relationships that never would be,
if grief hadn't invaded,
and took ahold of me.

What about these friendships,
built out of ache,
with those unafraid
of how my world did quake.

Beautiful souls.
Angels in flesh.
Beauty from ash.
Light in darkness.

It takes a different kind
to run into the fire.
To breathe life into someone
you didn't know prior.

I want to be that.
A light that shines through.
To pay it on forward.
Be a flesh angel –
to you.

The Day Will Come

There comes a day in your grief –

a day where you realize
you've stopped doing certain things.

Maybe you didn't cry today.

Maybe your person wasn't your first thought. Or your last.
Or every thought in-between.

Maybe you didn't get lost amongst their things today.

The cemetery – maybe you didn't go.

And at some point it will hit you.
Like a crushing wave, it will hit you.

You don't want to go a day without crying.

You don't want to start your day or end your day
without some thought of them.

You don't want any other thought in-between.

And immediately, you go lose yourself in their things.

You wrap your arms around a certain something
as if you're holding onto them.

"I'm so sorry," you whisper. "I'm so sorry."

Something about my grief that nobody knows…

That I don't want it to get lighter.
That the thought of it ever going just makes me grip tighter.

Yes, it was the unasked for guest.
Yes, it put me through the ringer
and every kind of test.
Yes, it was a hostile takeover
and I, its conquest.

But I sure don't want it to go.
Although it captured, and triumphed,
it no longer feels like a foe.

Grief has a space now in my home.
A seat at the table…
And freedom…
to roam.

It's wild how that happens ya know.
Whom you once begged to leave, you now plead to not go.

But I know that it will stay.
That I don't ever have to worry about it leaving one day.

And in this game of life,
where there is no guarantee…

That is a truth I can count on –
The grief… with me.

I Miss

I miss you. I miss me.

I miss what was,
what could've been,
what never will be.

I miss us. I miss them.

I miss wholeness, and fullness,
what we'll never be… again.

I miss the future.
The past.
Thinking present day struggles
one day would pass.

I miss effortlessness.
And simplicity.
I miss innocence.
And naivety.

I miss focus and structure.
And days of production.
I miss cyclical seasons,
likelihood and prediction.

I miss it all.
The way life should be.
How it would be…
if you were with me.

The Plan

His eyes saw you when you were formless.

All your days,
written in His book
and planned
before a single one of them
came to be.

Oh how I've wrestled with this.

2 years, 5 months, 24 days.

That was your planned
and written time.

All along,
He knew.

I say thank you and ask why all in one breath.

Your plan…
what was it?

Isn't the plan supposed to prosper and not harm?
Isn't is supposed to give hope and a future?

But what is both hope and a future if not Heaven?
Exactly where you are.

Perhaps He knew there was more harm for you,
for all of us,
if your days were ordained differently.

Perhaps the plan was this:

I am going to gift you to this family.
This lost family.

And I'm going to watch
as you wrap each one of them
around your tiny little finger,
and lead them all,
right back to me.

I am the way, the truth, and the life.
No one comes to the Father, except through me.

Perhaps He knew the only way
this lost family could be found
was through you.

Perhaps He knew
the only way
to give this family hope
and a future
was through you.

Perhaps His love for us is so great
He'll go to any extreme
to draw us to Him.

Perhaps He said, *Rescue them. Rescue them.*

Perhaps.

Thought you should know… When you lose a child at such a young age, you can't help but wonder what God's plan for them possibly could have been. 2 years old my girl was when she was taken home. 2 years old. To me, I always had this idea in my mind that my child's life would really begin when they left the nest, when they could spread their wings wide, and fly out into the big wide world on their own. But this poem highlights something else. Isn't God's plan for mankind Jesus? To have eternal life through belief in the One who can get us there. I find comfort in thinking that was Mallory's plan. To lead our family to Jesus, gifting us an eternity together that we maybe never would have if she didn't get there first. Maybe that was her purpose.

A Godly Conversation

"If God is in control of all things,
then He was in control of this too."

Yes, that is true.

"Then how can you say
He's a good God
if He let this happen to you."

Your question is fair.
I've asked it myself.
He could have intervened
or restored her to health.

The truth is,
I don't know why He allowed it.
Not from where I stand.

But you must always remember,
she was never even in my plan.

"Why is that important?
I'm not sure that I follow."

Well it's important because
He knew what I didn't know.

She was exactly what I needed.
His gift from up above.

He graced me with that child,
and her sweet, unconditional love.

That is why I trust Him.
He gave her to me.

While not in MY plan,
She was in HIS plan for me.

So clearly He knows better.
He knows what I know not.

Her life will always shape me,
whether she's here with me…
or not.

Dear Grief

Teach me again how to live.
How to live
with the force
of your ache.

Teach me again how to breathe.
How to breathe
with your weight
I can't shake.

Teach my heart how to beat.
How to pulse
through the burn
of your fire.

Teach my mind how to see.
How to view life
as a thing
to desire.

Teach me to rise with the clouds.
Teach me to dance in the rain.

Teach me to smile through tears.
And to do so without feeling shame.

Teach me to move with the stillness.
To step into the light of tomorrow.
Teach me to cut through the silence.
To sing - despite the sound of your sorrow.

Grief, teach me to grab life by the horns.
To take hold again of the reigns.

Grief, teach me to live to the fullest,
alongside you, for our days that remain.

Grief, I now just exist with your anguish.
Your torment tied into my soul.

Can you teach me a place of contentedness,
as you go with me wherever I go.

Grief, let's do this together.
Let's jointly soar to the sky.

Because we're partnered in this thing they call life.

And only you…
can teach me…
to fly.

The Miracle

Dear Griever

I challenge you to see your story as I do.

Each of us has a story of survival.
A tale of our own trauma.
An account of our continued existence.

We often climb up our own story mountain,
blinded to the themes in our story's arc.
We are unaware of the underlying currents,
that keep moving our story forward.

Themes like endurance,
courage and perseverance.

Currents like love, strength,
and heroism.

We can't usually see beyond our first plot twist.
The twist that changed the trajectory of our entire landscape,
turning our "feel good" story,
to one of survival.

We grievers are often left wondering,
"Why did my story need to be built upon suffering?"
"Why couldn't it be built upon a miracle?"

But what we don't realize is that there IS a miracle in our story.

You see, once upon a time, there was a soul who was shattered.
A soul that lost a world,
as they had always known it.

And every step of the climb in this altered reality,
brought with it a crossroads.
The path chosen,
key to their very survival.

Good versus evil.
Forgiveness versus revenge.
Love versus hate.
Giving up versus keeping on.

The invitation to give up and give in, oh so enticing.
The dark over light, oh so inviting.

But they didn't give up.
And they didn't give in.
Each step, the next right thing.

And you see,
if you tally up all those chosen paths,
the themes become crystal clear.

Endurance.
Courage.
Perseverance.
Love.
Strength.
Heroism.

Every griever has their own survival story, yes.
We have a trauma tale, oh yes.
But when we read between the lines,
when I… read between the lines,
I see the miracle in your story.
I can even see the miracle in mine.

We grievers, are the miracle.

If I Could Tell You Just One More Thing

If I could tell you just one more thing,
it would be how much I love you.
I love you as far as the east to the west.
And from here, to the shiny moon.
I don't know if you know this,
as you were taken way too soon.

If I could tell you just one more thing,
it's that you make me so damn proud.
You deserve to be celebrated.
Commemorated.
And spoken of out loud.
I don't know if you know this…
the extent of how damn proud.

If I could tell you just one more thing,
you're the greatest gift of my life.
Worth all of the heartache.
The undoing.
The difficulty,
and strife.
I don't know if you know this…
sweet treasure of my life.

If I could tell you just one more thing,
you are the sun to my sky.
The core of my universe.
And the apple to my eye.
I'm not sure you ever knew this…
brilliant light to my dark sky.

If I could tell you just one more thing,
you are the greatest of any surprise.
The most glorious of any rainbow.
The brightest star to my nighttime skies.
I'm not sure if you know this…
my beautiful and precious prize.

If I could tell you just one more thing,
I'd offer the deepest apology.
I'm sorry I didn't see death coming.
And I'm sorry I couldn't step in-between.
I wish that you could know this…
that I would have lured death to me.

If I could tell you just one more thing,
I'd whisper this to you.
A mother's love is so damn strong.
I would've given anything for you.

Oh how I wish that you could know this,
I would have given my life to you.

Yes, if I could tell you just one more thing,
I'd squeeze… all that… right in.

I'd tell you that you're everything
that makes a life worth living.

And any good that comes outta me,
well that's YOUR light, within.

Acknowledgments

Seeing this book in its completion is a bittersweet moment for me. Bitter, because there would be no book if there were still a sweet little girl here named Mallory. Bitter because an entire section would be missing if there were no pregnancy loss. And it goes without saying that I'd forego this accomplishment to have that little person back in my arms in a heartbeat. I'd forgo that entire section to have a baby in my arms. But the harsh reality is that both are not here, and that makes an accomplishment like this sacred to me. This book helps one child's memory to live on and gives voice to another kind of grief that too many women suffer alone.

This book would not be possible without the love and support of my family, friends, and community – all of whom continuously encourage me to keep sharing.

I'd like to thank my husband, Brian, for his faith in my ability to do this. His emotional backing is the reason I am able to. This is not just my life I'm sharing about. It is our life. He very easily – and understandably - could have preferred I privatize my grief. Not only did he not expect that of me, he encouraged me to delve even deeper, and for that, I am so grateful.

To my mother, Debra Heslin. Thank you for believing in me. Thank you for your help getting my writing out there. This book, like the other, would never have been published if it weren't for your commitment to making sure it did. I am so grateful.

To my children, Brandon and Miranda – you are the most resilient children I know. You bring so much purpose to my life. I know one day you will be able to read through these pages and fully grasp all you have seen and been through. Your unwavering trust and faith in God, and not ever wanting to be the reason you were steered away, has kept me on His path. Thank you for being the best little disciples.

Finally, to my @Grief – The Write Way community - you have become home base for me. You're the place where I trial my writing, process my loss, and feel safe to share. It was through sharing with you that I realized I wanted to compile all of this poetry together in one place. Out of you grew one book, and now another. Thank you to all who make up that special community.

About the Author

My name is Cherie Fertitta Pinheiro. This may be the most unusual "About the Author" you've ever read because I'm not here to give a synopsis of my accomplishments or credentials like most others do. It's not that I wouldn't want to – it's simply because I don't have any.

I'll be honest and tell you: there's nothing special about me. I'm not an accredited writer. I've journaled at different stages of my life to process and release big emotions, but I've rarely shared those writings with anyone. That is, until my world imploded and I lost my youngest child.

My loss is my credentials. My children are my accomplishments. My identity has been wrapped up in my children for over a decade now. I've spent the past 11 years being a stay-at-home mom to three beautiful children: Brandon, age 11; Miranda, age 9; and Mallory, forever 2-1/2. But now I have a new headline on my motherhood resume: grieving mother.

I am a grieving mother. And I'm pretty sure nothing qualifies someone more to write about this kind of loss than a person who daily breathes that exact air. Writing has been my lifeline throughout this journey. I've felt led to share it in hopes of supporting anyone else who knows grief as intimately as I do, but who may not have the words to describe it.

My first book, *I Will Speak of You,* was to serve that purpose, and so is this new one. Let my words be your words. They say it takes a village, and grief is no different. It is my privilege to be a part of yours.

Made in United States
Orlando, FL
27 November 2025